TODAY'S TREATMENT: 2

TODAY'S TREATMENT: 2

Articles published in
the *British Medical Journal*

Published by the British Medical Association
Tavistock Square, London WC1H 9JR

ERRATA
Page 78 line 37: the dose should read "as little as 0.0625 daily".

ISBN 0 7279 0025 0

Made and printed in England by
The Devonshire Press
Barton Road, Torquay

Preface

by the Editor
British Medical Journal

This is the second volume of *Today's Treatment*, collected from articles published in the *BMJ* in 1976 and 1977. Like its predecessor, it contains broad reviews of the spectrum of treatments available for different conditions. These assessments are likely to remain valid and of practical help for several years, and the series is intended to provide a working manual for doctors in clinical practice.

Keeping abreast of recent advances is a recurrent problem for all clinicians: in comparing the new preparations with the best of the older drugs and treatments *Today's Treatment* achieves, we believe, a reasonable compromise between innovation and conservatism.

STEPHEN LOCK
1977

Contents

Endocrine and metabolic diseases

Diseases of the cardiovascular system

Diseases of the alimentary system

Endocrine and metabolic diseases

Adrenal diseases

G M BESSER, W J JEFFCOATE

Each adrenal gland is composed of two embryologically, anatomically, and functionally distinct parts—the medulla and cortex. Diseases of the adrenal medulla are confined to the development of tumours, which may be benign or malignant and which may or may not secrete catecholamines (table). There is no recognised clinical syndrome involving underactivity of the adrenal medulla. Diseases of the adrenal cortex on the other hand may be characterised by either over- or under-production of its hormones: glucocorticoids, mineralocorticoids, or sex steroids. When a hormone (or hormones) is produced in excess, it may derive from an adenoma, carcinoma, or generalised hyperplasia of the glands. When hormone production is inadequate, it may be the result of congenital defects, organic disease of the gland, or impaired adreno-corticotrophic hormone (ACTH) or renin production.

Diseases of the adrenal medulla

Tumour	Cell type	Age	Note
Sympathoblastoma	Sympathogone	Infancy	Highly malignant
Neuroblastoma	Sympathoblast	Childhood	Highly malignant, may secrete catecholamines
Ganglioneuroma	Ganglion cells	Young adults	Benign or malignant
Phaeochromocytoma	Chromaffin cells	Adults	Benign or malignant, secrete catecholamines

DISEASES OF THE ADRENAL MEDULLA

Poorly differentiated tumours

The sympathoblastoma of infancy is highly malignant and treatment is almost uniformly unsuccessful. Neuroblastomas tend to occur in older children. They also are highly malignant, although a combination of surgery and radiotherapy is rewarded by apparent cure in 10%. Neuroblastomas may secrete catecholamines. Ganglioneuromas are rare tumours that occur in young adults. They may be benign or malignant.

Phaeochromocytomas

About 10% of phaeochromocytomas are bilateral and about 10% are not in the adrenal at all: they may be anywhere in the distribution of sympathetic neural tissue. When extra-adrenal they are most commonly found in the sympathetic chain, the bladder wall, or para-aortic bodies of Zuckerkandl; 10% are malignant.

Because of the excessive secretion of catecholamines from these tumours hypertensive crises and arrhythmias may occur. These attacks may, however, be entirely or largely blocked by treatment with alpha- and beta-adrenoceptor blocking drugs. Oral propranolol (40–80 mg eight hourly) and oral phenoxybenzamine (10–20 mg eight hourly) are recommended for those patients in whom removal of the tumour is either impossible or deferred. Care should be exercised in using these drugs together since hypotension may follow. They should preferably be first introduced while the patient is in hospital. If a patient has the rare form of phaeochromocytoma that is characterised by hypotensive attacks propranolol should be given alone.

Hypertensive crises and arrhythmias may occur also during investigative procedures such as arteriography, during abdominal surgery of any kind, and during labour. Preparation with alpha- and beta-blocking agents for these and for removal of the adrenal tumour itself must therefore always be performed. Daily infusions of phenoxybenzamine should be given for three days—in a dose of 1 mg/kg body weight in 250 ml of 5% dextrose infused over one hour. Propranolol is given by mouth, 40 mg eight hourly, over the same period—the first dose being given after the first infusion of phenoxybenzamine.[1]

Profound hypotensive collapse may follow removal of a phaeochromocytoma. Patients with these tumours have a low plasma volume as a result of tonic vasoconstriction, and removal of the tumour is followed by widespread vasodilatation and the blood pressure falls. The preoperative preparation with phenoxybenzamine and propranolol allows expansion of the blood volume before surgery and prevents collapse. Nevertheless, adequate volumes of blood must be available for transfusion if necessary.

DISEASES OF THE ADRENAL CORTEX

Cushing's syndrome

The causes of Cushing's syndrome fall into two main groups: (*a*) ACTH-dependent, due to excessive secretion of ACTH from the pituitary (Cushing's disease), or from non-endocrine hormone secreting tumours (the ectopic ACTH syndrome), or due to treatment with exogenous ACTH; and (*b*) non-ACTH-dependent—benign or malignant adrenocortical tumours, or treatment with exogenous corticosteroids.

Pituitary-dependent bilateral adrenal hyperplasia (*Cushing's disease*)—The logical treatment of Cushing's disease is to remove the source of

ACTH production from the pituitary. Unfortunately, this logical approach is not always possible. External irradiation of the pituitary gland produces cure in 25% and improvement in only a further 20%. The pituitary may be attacked by external irradiation using protons, implantation of radioactive yttrium or gold seeds, cryosurgery, and microdissection of the pituitary by the transphenoidal route; each has its advocates but no technique is in widespread use. Pituitary microdissection may well prove to be the treatment of choice in the future for good results have been claimed; it is sometimes possible to recognise and remove a small adenoma with only minimal disturbance to the rest of the gland. At the moment the technical expertise required for this operation is not widely available and experience is limited.

The main problem of conventional external irradiation is the delay of up to four years which may occur before it is fully effective. Often the patient with Cushing's disease is severely ill and this delay is unacceptable. This is why the combination of pituitary irradiation and bilateral adrenalectomy remains the treatment of choice in most centres. If a patient has an adrenalectomy but no irradiation he runs the risk of developing hyperpigmentation and enlargement of the pituitary fossa (Nelson's syndrome). This may be prevented by conventional external pituitary irradiation (4500 rads over four to five weeks) given within two months of adrenalectomy. After adrenalectomy patients must receive replacement treatment as for Addison's disease (see below).

We now use metyrapone for the long-term control of Cushing's disease. Its use is associated with a rapid clinical improvement that is maintained for long periods (one patient has been followed for four years). When used in combination with pituitary irradiation it provides a reversible "medical adrenalectomy" that controls the disease until the radiotherapy is effective. This regimen, however, has not been used for long enough for us to be sure of its overall long-term efficacy. Metyrapone lowers the production of cortisol in the adrenocortical cells by blocking enzymes controlling its synthesis. The dose chosen has to be individually tailored to each patient; it varies from 250 mg twice daily to 1 g six hourly. An average plasma fluorogenic corticosteroid level of 300–380 nmol/l (11–14 μg/100 ml) throughout the day is the aim since this will be associated with a normal 24-hour cortisol production rate.

Rarely, metyrapone will not control cortisol production fully and then aminoglutethimide may be added in a dose of 250 or 500 mg eight hourly. It is, however, much more toxic than metyrapone. Because of the danger of adrenocortical insufficiency this "medical adrenalectomy" should be confined to those centres with facilities for frequent and rapid measurement of plasma cortisol. Undoubtedly, however, surgery may be avoided in many patients as a result of this treatment.

Adrenal diseases

Ectopic ACTH syndrome

The management of ectopic ACTH syndrome is similar to that of Cushing's disease. If the source of ACTH can be removed, it should be done. Alternatively, the primary lesion may respond to irradiation or chemotherapy. The greatly raised cortisol levels in blood may be controlled using metyrapone as in Cushing's disease. Often these patients are very sensitive to this drug and close monitoring of plasma corticosteroid levels throughout the day is necessary until the effective dose is reached. Some cover their patients with prednisolone (5 mg two to three times daily) or dexamethasone (0·5 mg two to three times daily) until the therapeutically adequate dose of metyrapone is reached but doing this may worsen the Cushingoid state. In these often very ill patients average daily plasma corticosteroid levels of about 552 nmol/l (20 μg/100 ml) should be the aim of treatment. Spironolactone should not be used to treat the hypokalaemia since it interferes with the usual fluorescent assay of plasma cortisol. Triamterene (50 to 100 mg three times daily) is better. Oral potassium supplements are also necessary at least initially.

Adrenocortical adenoma—Treatment of adrenocortical adenoma is by excision. As with phaeochromocytoma, the tumours are bilateral in about 10% of cases and unless the side they are on can be precisely determined it is usual to recommend exploration of both glands. This is a big operation usually performed through an anterior approach and is associated with considerable morbidity. The risks are high because the untreated patient may be hypertensive and diabetic, has a bruising tendency, and has poor wound healing. Chronic potassium depletion may be present. Attempts may be made to localise the tumour before surgery. Plain abdominal *x*-ray examination or intravenous pyelography may help if the tumour is large.

Selective adrenal vein catheterisation may be used, but the most promising technique is the recently developed one of adrenal scanning with radioactively labelled iodocholesterol. With information from these investigations the surgeon may opt for the quicker, safer operation—exploring only one side through a loin incision.

As in Cushing's disease we also use metyrapone when preparing patients with adrenal tumours for operation. If a patient receives this drug for three months before surgery many features of this disease, including hypertension, diabetes, heart failure, plethora, and obesity will improve; the operation is easier and morbidity is considerably reduced.

Adrenocortical carcinoma—Similar principles relate to managing adrenal carcinoma. While leisurely preoperative preparation is obviously inappropriate, preparation with metyrapone need not be omitted altogether. Another drug that may be used is mitotane (o-p′-DDD), which was originally discovered as a contaminant of DDT and which destroys both normal and malignant adrenocortical cells. Its use provides palliative control of the carcinoma and metastases for long periods. Eventually, however, the tumour escapes from its control. The doses used are often large (between 10 and 20 g in divided doses) and it may cause considerable gastrointestinal side effects.

Iatrogenic Cushing's syndrome—Withdrawal of the corticosteroids should be performed with care since it is well known that their use suppresses the hypothalamic-pituitary-adrenal axis. Any prolonged suppression that occurs is at the level of the hypothalamus or pituitary, and not the adrenal since adrenal atrophy quickly recovers. Hence a patient who has been withdrawn from steroids and is shown to have a normal cortisol response to ACTH need not necessarily have a normal cortisol response to stress.

Hyperaldosteronism

Primary hyperaldosteronism (Conn's syndrome) may result from either adenoma or hyperplasia of the zona glomerulosa. It may be that when there is hyperplasia the hyperaldosteronism is not primary but secondary to some unrecognised adrenal-stimulating factor.

Adenomas occur more commonly on the left side, but they may be bilateral. As in other types of adrenal tumour it is conventional to explore both sides through an anterior approach although use of the localising techniques described above may allow the surgeon to explore only one side. Malignancy of these tumours is rare.

Spironolactone competitively blocks the renal effect of circulating aldosterone. In this condition the doses need to be high (100–400 mg daily) but it is not necessary to divide the dose. It may be used to control the disease before surgery; preoperative preparation is recommended since the patients are usually severely potassium-depleted and hypertensive. Indeed, spironolactone controls the condition so effectively that it may be used for long-term control if for any reason surgery is contraindicated. In most cases oral potassium supplements should be used in addition to spironolactone, at least until the patient has been stabilised.

After removal of an aldosterone-secreting adenoma there may be temporary rebound hyperkalaemia resulting from suppression of the remaining normal zona glomerulosa. Fludrocortisone may then be required temporarily in doses of 0·05 mg on alternate days to 0·1 mg daily.

Renin-secreting tumours of the kidney, haemangiopericytomas, are a rare cause of secondary hyperaldosteronism. The patients present with hypertension, hypokalaemia, and bilateral hyperplasia of the zona glomerulosa with hyperaldosteronism. The condition may be cured by removing the tumour.

Adrenal diseases

Virilising and feminising tumours

Both virilising and feminising tumours are uncommon, particularly the latter. After the diagnosis is made treatment is by excision.

Adrenocortical insufficiency

There may be deficient secretion of glucocorticoids, of mineralocorticoids, or of both. The causes of adrenal insufficiency are: (*a*) primary: autoimmune, tuberculosis, carcinomatosis, amyloidosis and other infiltrations, haemochromatosis, postadrenalectomy; and (*b*) secondary: ACTH deficiency and renin deficiency. When there is organic disease of the adrenals or after adrenalectomy there is deficient secretion of both cortisol and aldosterone and both must be replaced. ACTH deficiency, on the other hand, does not lead to a fall in aldosterone secretion and only cortisol replacement is needed. Congenital enzyme defects occur in the group of diseases known as congenital adrenal hyperplasia. These are dealt with below. Isolated mineralocorticoid deficiency is diagnosed only rarely, but its true incidence is unknown. It is probably always the result of diminished renin secretion.

The traditional replacement treatment for cortisol deficiency in the past has been cortisone acetate (such as 25 mg in the morning and 12·5 mg in the evening), but this drug is now being abandoned in most centres since it is irregularly absorbed from the bowel and because it has to be converted to hydrocortisone in the body before becoming active. Hydrocortisone should be used instead in doses of about 20 mg on waking and 10 mg in the evening but the dose should be tailored to each individual patient. This may be done by measuring the levels of cortisol in the plasma throughout the day—the peak after the morning oral dose should be 690–960 nmol/l (25–35 μg/100 ml); before the evening dose the levels should be 170–270 nmol/l (6–10 μg/100 ml) and after the evening dose peak levels should not exceed 690 nmol/l (25 μg/100 ml). Prednisolone (5 mg and 2·5 mg) and dexamethasone (0·5 mg and 0·25 mg) may be used instead of hydrocortisone, but their levels cannot easily be measured in the plasma.

When patients are receiving long-term replacement treatment with prednisolone, hydrocortisone, or dexamethasone, the morning dose should be taken as soon as the patient awakes. The evening dose should be taken at about 6 pm. If it is taken later the patient may be troubled by wakefulness or nocturia. Every patient should wear a bracelet or necklet with the diagnosis and reference number engraved upon it.* If he suffers any injury or illness other than a slight head cold he should double the dose of his tablets. If he has a more severe illness or one in which he is unable to take his tablets for any other reason the doctor

* Obtainable from Medic-Alert Foundation, 9 Hanover Street, London W1R 9HF.

should be called and he should be given intramuscular hydrocortisone (50 to 100 mg every six to eight hours). We give our patients a supply of parenteral hydrocortisone to keep in the house in case of emergency.

Mineralocorticoid deficiency is usually replaced with fludrocortisone. The drug is given daily or on alternate days in doses of 0·05 to 0·1 mg. Overdose is uncommon but is attended by clinical evidence of fluid overload. It is not necessary to increase the dose of fludrocortisone during intercurrent illness.

Congenital adrenal hyperplasia

Congenital adrenal hyperplasia results from the congenital deficiency of one or more enzymes needed for the normal formation of adrenal corticosteroids. The commonest deficiency is that of the 21-hydroxylase enzyme. As a result of the corticosteroid deficiency, ACTH secretion increases, the gland becomes hyperplastic, and the precursors of hydrocortisone accumulate and are converted to androgenic steroids. Girls are therefore virilised at birth; boys have precocious sexual development in infancy. Both boys and girls are tall and strong as young children, but their epiphyses fuse early (if untreated) and they are stunted as adults. Treatment is simple and consists of providing corticosteroids that they lack. Less often the sepatients are also "salt-losers" at birth—that is, they cannot conserve sodium efficiently. They need added salt and fludrocortisone in addition to glucocorticoid. The circadian rhythm of ACTH secretion has its nadir at the normal time of retiring and its peak in the early morning. In congenital adrenal hyperplasia the object of treatment is to suppress endogenous ACTH as fully as possible, and it has been found that this is best achieved by giving the larger part of the corticosteroid dose at the nadir. This is why these patients should be given two thirds of the total daily dose of prednisolone or dexamethasone last thing at night and the remainder on waking. On this regimen urinary 17-oxosteroids should be less than 10 μmol/24 h (3 mg/24 h), urine pregnanetriol less than 7 μmol/24 h (2 mg/24 h), plasma cortisol less than 110 nmol/l (4 μg/100 ml), and plasma ACTH suppressed. The total dose in children depends on body weight and in adolescents and adults is 7·5 mg per day of prednisolone.

The condition of congenital adrenal hyperplasia is nowadays usually recognised at birth. If lifelong replacement is started immediately in these babies their subsequent development will be almost entirely normal, the only exception being that some girls may require minor plastic surgery to their external genitalia.

REFERENCES

1 Ross, E J, *et al*, *British Medical Journal*, 1967, **1**, 191.

Pituitary diseases

J A STRONG

The scope for better management of patients with pituitary disorders has been greatly improved in recent years by a series of advances. Developments in protein chemistry have provided an almost complete range of natural or synthetic replacements for the hormones of the pituitary gland, available for use when needed. Some of the hypothalamic hormones have been identified, synthesised, and made available for clinical application. Methods of controlling excessive secretion of pituitary hormones have been improved. Hormone assays are now widely available and may be used to define precisely the nature and extent of disordered pituitary function, as well as to monitor the response to treatment. The laboratory service for these assays has recently been established in Britain on a regional and national basis in the National Health Service or university-supported establishments. A commercial hormone assay service is also available and can provide almost any test likely to be needed.

The relevance of the close anatomical and functional relationship between the hypothalamus and the pituitary gland has received fresh emphasis with the introduction into clinical practice of hypothalamic hormones (see table). The first of these was thyrotrophin-releasing hormone followed by gonadotrophin-releasing hormone (GRH) and more recently growth hormone release inhibiting hormone (somatostatin). Several drugs also have analogous effects on this system—for example, bromocriptine, clomiphene, levodopa, and the phenothiazines.

Effective management of pituitary diseases requires a grasp of all these considerations and of the opportunity that these developments provide for full correction of disordered function.

Pituitary disease may present in many ways. Endocrine effects from hypersecretion of a single hormone, usually growth hormone (GH) or adrenocorticotrophic hormone (ACTH), may predominate. Occasionally the output of more than one hormone may be increased. On the other hand, partial or complete failure to secrete one pituitary hormone or more may be found, or hypersecretion of one hormone—for example, GH—may be associated with failure to secrete some or all of the remainder. This potential variety of change helps to emphasise the value of hormone assays in management. In addition to disorders of function, structural changes in the gland, as a result of trauma, infection, infarction, and tumour, may in turn produce their own specific clinical features.

PITUITARY TUMOURS

Some of the visual symptoms associated with a pituitary tumour, most commonly a change in acuity, are readily recognised by patients: nevertheless, they may easily overlook a visual field defect large enough to be detected by confrontation. Features such as these are an urgent indication for neurosurgical advice and in most instances for decompression of the optic chiasma. The choice of procedure may lie between a craniotomy and a transfrontal approach to the sella turcica or an extracranial path by the trans-sphenoidal route may be chosen.

Many surgeons advise a course of radiotherapy after operation on chromophobe or eosinophil adenomas of the pituitary gland to suppress any tumour tissue that may remain. Others prefer to avoid an open operative procedure, particularly if the visual fields are intact, and instead attempt to destroy the tumour either by irradiation from external sources or by implanting sources of radiation such as yttrium-90 within the pituitary tumour. This may be done through a cannula inserted under radiographic control through the nose into the sella turcica. A similar route may be used to insert a probe carrying a cryosurgical device which allows the operator to destroy, by the application of cold, the tissue surrounding the tip of the probe. Thus a wide range of procedures is available for the treatment of pituitary tumours; the choice in each patient will depend on many factors, including the techniques available in any particular centre.

Abnormalities of hormone secretion

A pituitary tumour must be treated on its merits, both as a surgical problem of space-occupation with potential pressure effects and as a medical problem of hypersecretion or secretory failure, with the need to suppress or replace. Secretion of pituitary hormones may be abnormal because of disorders primarily in the gland itself, or the abnormality may derive from disordered function in the hypothalamus affecting the secretion of releasing or inhibitory hormones.

PITUITARY HYPERSECRETION

Of the seven hormones produced by the anterior lobe of the normal pituitary gland, excessive secretion of three only—namely, GH, ACTH, and prolactin—is likely to need intervention. Hypersecretion of GH is usually associated with acromegaly and an eosinophil adenoma of the pituitary gland. Persistent hypersecretion in these circumstances may be associated with diabetes mellitus and hypertension, in addition to the other features of acromegaly. There are good reasons, therefore, for suppressing GH secretion when assays show this to be persistent and excessive. Destruction of the tumour is usually attempted, but there is often some residual hypersecretion. Bromocriptine may be used as a

Pituitary hormones and hypothalamic hormones or factors that control production of the former. Secretion of pituitary hormones without a specific endocrine gland as target appears to be controlled by both releasing and release-inhibiting hormones formed in the hypothalamus. Hypothalamic factors are referred to as hormones when their chemical structure has been determined

Hypothalamic hormones and factors	Abbreviation	Pituitary hormone	Abbreviation	Target
Thyrotrophin releasing hormone	TRH	Thyroid stimulating hormone (thyrotrophin)	TSH	Thyroid gland
Corticotrophin releasing factor	CRF	Adrenocorticotrophic hormone	ACTH	Adrenal cortex
Gonadotrophin releasing hormone	GRH	Luteinising hormone	LH	Ovary
		Interstitial cell-stimulating hormone	ICSH	Testis
		Follicle-stimulating hormone	FSH	Ovary, Testis
Prolactin releasing factor	PRF	Prolactin		Breast
Prolactin inhibiting factor	PIF	Prolactin		Breast
Growth hormone releasing factor	GHRF	Growth hormone	GH	Numerous
Growth hormone release inhibiting hormone (somatostatin)	GHRIH	Growth hormone	GH	Numerous
MSH release and inhibiting factors		Melanocyte stimulating hormone	MSH	Melanocytes

supplement to surgery or radiotherapy to suppress secretion of GH in acromegaly, but the drug is still undergoing clinical trials.

Pituitary basophilism with a raised output of ACTH is responsible for many cases of Cushing's syndrome. Pituitary basophil adenomas are usually so small as to be undetectable by the usual methods and bilateral adrenalectomy is still appropriate. In some patients treated in this way, the pituitary basophil adenoma may grow slowly over several years until it becomes clinically apparent, when it would merit treatment if it is producing local pressure effects. Sometimes persistent hypersecretion of ACTH and the melanocyte stimulating hormone are associated, so that the patient becomes inordinately pigmented as in Addison's disease, in spite of adequate replacement treatment with corticosteroids (Nelson's syndrome).

Excessive secretion of prolactin is usually recognised because it is associated with galactorrhoea, though the hormone may be circulating in excess without this feature. There are many potential causes of galactorrhoea but a principal mechanism appears to be failure to maintain an appropriate level of production of the hypothalamic prolactin release inhibiting factor. An important though rare cause is a craniopharyngioma, blocking the pathway between the hypothalamus and the pituitary gland, but destructive lesions of the hypothalamus, other endocrine disorders, and some drugs may be responsible. Bromocriptine is even more effective in suppressing secretion of prolactin than it is in suppressing GH in acromegaly. Hyperprolactinaemia may accompany secondary amenorrhoea and cause infertility that can be corrected by bromocriptine. Indeed, some patients under treatment with bromocriptine for acromegaly and for galactorrhoea have proved surprisingly fertile.

HYPOPITUITARISM

The development and clinical application of a comprehensive range of assays for pituitary hormones make it more logical to describe pituitary failure in terms of the precise nature and extent of the hormone deficit rather than as a series of clinical syndromes, a concept more appropriate to a discussion on diagnosis than on treatment.

Growth hormone

Although failure of GH secretion is a feature of many patients with pituitary disease, the only clinical condition in which the use of this scarce and expensive hormone may be justified at present is in dwarfs who are shown by assays to be GH deficient. Species specificity and the need therefore to use material of human origin, coupled with the scarcity of therapeutic preparations, have restricted the use of this material. Where the conditions for use are fulfilled, however, and the child is aged under about 12, successful growth has been achieved. Supplies of growth hormone in Britain are distributed by the Medical Research Council for use in carefully selected cases.

Thyrotrophin

Hypothyroidism is a common complication of pituitary insufficiency, but such patients should be treated with thyroxine, rather than attempting to use thyroid-stimulating hormone as a substitute. When starting treatment it is important to ensure that adequate corticosteroid replacement treatment has been given before initiating treatment with thyroxine; otherwise acute adrenal insufficiency or coma may be precipitated. Conventional doses up to 0·2 mg daily of thyroxine may be needed in an adult.

Corticotrophin

Failure of ACTH secretion is the most important endocrine defect in hypopituitarism because it is potentially the most lethal. The need for replacement treatment is judged on the evidence of adrenocortical insufficiency, which may be shown to be reversible by injecting ACTH. In view of the expense, the need to give ACTH or one of the synthetic analogues by injection, and the less predictable plasma levels of corticosteroids that may be achieved in this way, ACTH is seldom used in treating hypopituitarism. Corticosteroids are usually given, and prednisolone or prednisone are to be preferred to cortisol or cortisone, since oedema is more likely to occur with the two latter steroids. Doses cannot be predicted precisely for every individual, but an average requirement would be 5 mg of prednisolone in the morning and 2·5 mg in the evening.

The usual precautions about increasing the dose of steroid two-, three-, or four-fold in the face of the stress of infection, injury, or operation—if necessary substituting a steroid given by injection—must be emphasised to the patient, who should be urged always to carry a card or to wear a bracelet indicating his requirements.

Gonadotrophins

Initiation of gonadal function in the adolescent of both sexes and its maintenance in the adult depends upon the stimulus provided to the ovary and testis by the pituitary gonadotrophins follicle-stimulating hormone (FSH) and luteinising hormone (LH) (interstitial cell-stimulating hormone). Production of these hormones by the pituitary gland depends in turn on the hypothalamic releasing hormone gonadotrophin releasing hormone (GRH) (luteinising hormone releasing hormone). The clinical features will vary according to the time of life at which hypothalamopituitary failure of gonadotrophin secretion develops. A late onset of puberty in either sex may cause much anxiety to patients and parents alike, and it may sometimes be reassuring to both to exclude pituitary disease by showing that pituitary function is normal. In most forms of pituitary disease with failure of hormone production, gonadotrophin secretion is usually the first to cease. Primary or secondary amenorrhoea may therefore be relatively early features of pituitary failure. In men, hypogonadism with failure to develop or maintain secondary sexual characteristics, impotence, or occasionally infertility may call for treatment.

In secondary gonadal insufficiency there is seldom any justification for attempting to treat this deficiency with pituitary hormones, and almost all the advantages lie with replacement treatment using gonadal hormones. In the female, ovarian hormone replacement treatment may be needed occasionally, and for this purpose numerous preparations of oestrogens and progestogens are available. A suitable combination is provided by many varieties of the contraceptive pill.

For the male, there are several methods available to replace androgen secretion. Fluoxymesterone may be taken by mouth, and in doses of 5–20 mg daily it is usually satisfactory. The dose should never exceed 20 mg/day. Many long-acting preparations of testosterone, which may be given conveniently at intervals of one to two weeks by intramuscular injection, are also available. Fused pellets of testosterone, each with 200 mg of the androgen, may be implanted subcutaneously through a cannula under the skin of the anterior abdominal wall. Five pellets usually provide adequate androgen for six to nine months.

When infertility in the female has been shown to be due to pituitary or hypothalamic disorder and not to ovarian disease there are several methods available for promoting ovulation. It is, of course, essential that the man should have been shown by seminal analysis to be potentially fertile before embarking on treatment to promote ovulation.

Treatment with clomiphene, given in courses of 50 mg twice daily for five days, may be followed by ovulation. GRH is under trial at present with similar objectives in mind. When the pituitary gland has been shown to be incapable of responding adequately to GRH or clomiphene, a suitable mixed preparation of FSH and LH (Pergonal), obtained from human menopausal urine, has been used successfully to treat failure of ovulation, and purer preparations of gonadotrophin, extracted from human pituitary glands, have also been effective. These preparations of gonadotrophins should only be used when facilities for monitoring the ovarian response by plasma assays of oestrogens and progesterone or by urinary oestrogen and pregnanediol assays are available.

Hormone treatment for male infertility needs full assessment of the patient with sperm counts before this is undertaken. The value of clomiphene and of gonadotrophins is being investigated.

Pituitary diseases

PANHYPOPITUITARISM

Panhypopituitarism is usually reserved for patients with complete failure of all the functions of the anterior lobe of the pituitary gland. They need replacement treatment with corticosteroids and thyroxine, and men may need androgen treatment. If they go unrecognised, stop their treatment, suffer an injury or a severe infection, or undergo an operation without their dose of corticosteroid being increased temporarily three- or four-fold they may lapse into coma, sometimes with hypothermia which may be rapidly fatal. In such a crisis they will need a full regimen of intravenous fluids and electrolyte replacement. Intravenous hydrocortisone should be given as an initial bolus of 100 mg, followed by infusion of 100 mg four-hourly, and antibiotics for any accompanying infection. Thyroxine replacement treatment is usually less urgent.

DIABETES INSIPIDUS

Loss of function of the posterior lobe of the pituitary gland and its connection with the hypothalamus characterises diabetes insipidus. But it may also be associated with damage to the anterior lobe of the pituitary gland. The condition, however, may develop after operations on or near the hypophysis, sometimes transiently and without evidence of damage to the function of the anterior lobe of the pituitary gland.

If the neurohypophysis is totally incapable of producing vasopressin the most satisfactory treatment, until recently, has been with pitressin tannate in oil, 5 units on alternate evenings by subcutaneous injection. Precautions were needed to ensure that the hormone reached the syringe and the patient. If the response failed to persist for a full 48 hours, supplements of lypressin could be given by nasal spray every few hours until the next injection was due. Pitressin tannate in oil, however, has now been withdrawn from the market. A new synthetic analogue of vasopressin—namely, desmopressin—has recently been marketed. This drug is very effective, the response lasting 12–24 hours after each nasal instillation, but the treatment will cost about £1 daily compared with about 5p using pitressin tannate in oil.

Alternative methods of controlling diabetes insipidus successfully, provided the patient can secrete some vasopressin, include the administration of chlorpropamide, 100–250 mg daily; clofibrate, 1 g daily; or carbamazepine, 100–400 mg daily. Thiazide diuretics—for example, bendrofluazide 5 mg daily—may also be effective by itself or in combination with some of the oral preparations already mentioned. Potassium supplements should be given if oral diuretics are used.

Most functions of the pituitary gland can now be replaced when the need arises. The means are available, and they should be used with monitoring services to ensure that the response is adequate but is not overdone.

Treatment of thyroid disease

D C EVERED

HYPERTHYROIDISM AND GRAVES'S DISEASE

Hyperthyroidism is a potentially serious condition and therefore merits treatment. Three specific methods of treatment are available: antithyroid drugs, partial thyroidectomy, and radioactive iodine.

Antithyroid drugs

It is possible to interfere pharmacologically with each stage of thyroid hormone synthesis, release, and transport. The usual drugs, however, are either inhibitors of organification (thionamides) or less frequently inhibitors of iodide transport (potassium perchlorate). Iodides, lithium compounds, and beta-adrenergic blockers have also been used, although the last group probably has no direct action upon the thyroid.

Thionamides—The major thionamide is carbimazole, which interferes with organification. Propylthiouracil may also inhibit the peripheral monodeiodination of thyroxine, but there is no good evidence that this action contributes to its therapeutic effect in man. Hyperthyroidism may be controlled in all patients with adequate doses of thionamides, but these drugs have a short half life and are usually administered in divided doses, although the necessity for doing so is disputed. The initial dose of carbimazole is 10–15 mg every six hours. A biochemical response is seen within one to two weeks, although the clinical response takes longer. The dose may be reduced and adjusted on the basis of clinical and biochemical observations as the hyperthyroidism comes under control. The alternative course is to maintain a full blocking dose of carbimazole and add 0·15 mg thyroxine to the patient's medication when the hyperthyroidism is under control. This latter procedure has the advantage that fluctuations in the patient's clinical state are avoided as the dose is progressively adjusted. Hypersensitivity reactions and agranulocytosis may occur but are rare with carbimazole. Propylthiouracil or methylthiouracil may be used as alternatives if hypersensitivity to carbimazole occurs. The initial dosage of these drugs is 300–400 mg daily.

Potassium perchlorate—This agent interferes with iodide transport and should only be used in patients who have developed hypersensitivity to the thionamides, since there is a higher risk of blood dyscrasias with this drug. The initial dose is 200 mg every six hours. Patients receiving perchlorate should not be given iodide since too much iodide will overcome the inhibition of transport.

Treatment of thyroid disease

Iodides—The actions of iodides on the thyroid are complex. Their use in the preparation of the patient for thyroidectomy has now been superseded by the combined use of carbimazole and thyroxine. The sole remaining use for iodides is in the management of thyroid crisis. The most suitable preparation is potassium iodide tablets (60 mg), although the traditional Lugol's iodine may be used.

Lithium compounds—Lithium compounds reduce the synthesis of thyroid hormone and also block hormone release. They have major metabolic and endocrine effects unrelated to the thyroid in addition to their other toxic effects. There is no justification for their use since safer and more specific drug treatments are available.

Beta-adrenergic blockers—Several clinical features of hyperthyroidism may be attributed to increased adrenergic activity. These effects will be improved by beta-blocking agents. There is no justification for using these drugs routinely since specific agents that control *all* the features of hyperthyroidism are available. The major use of beta-blockers, as an adjunct to other measures, is in the management of arrhythmias or in impending or actual thyroid crisis to minimise the cardiovascular effects of preformed hormone. The only beta-blocker that should be used for this purpose is propranolol since other preparations have intrinsic sympathomimetic activity.

Partial thyroidectomy

Partial thyroidectomy generally provides the most certain method of eliminating hyperthyroidism and goitre. There is also growing evidence that this procedure has a major effect on the immunological disturbances of Graves's disease. Surgery should never be performed in the unprepared patient. Preparation should be carried out with carbimazole to render the patient euthyroid and with thyroxine to eliminate the risk of thyroid-stimulating hormone stimulation of the blocked gland as described above.

Surgery should reduce the thyroid mass sufficiently to cure the hyperthyroidism but leave sufficient secretory tissue for the patient's needs. This is not always achieved. The incidence of hypothyroidism has been reported to lie at 3–35% and recurrent hyperthyroidism at 1·2–28%. Many factors play a part in these wide variations, including remnant size, the degree of lymphocytic infiltration of the gland, the extent of thyroid regeneration, the alteration in immunological status, and the precision of the diagnostic techniques used to identify abnormalities of thyroid function. The other main complications of thyroid surgery are hypoparathyroidism, recurrent laryngeal palsy, and thyroid crisis.

Radioiodine treatment

Radioiodine treatment was first introduced in 1942. It is almost invariably carried out using ^{131}I (early studies suggest that ^{125}I treatment has no appreciable advantage). This treatment is convenient for the patient, and early fears that there might be an increased frequency of thyroid carcinoma, leukaemia, or congenital abnormalities in the children of patients have been proved groundless. Radioiodine is generally reserved for patients over 40 and should never be given during pregnancy.

The administration of radioiodine may be followed by a transient increase in thyroid size and a release of preformed hormone into the circulation. Neither of these events is usually associated with clinical problems, although the latter may exacerbate an arrhythmia in a severely hyperthyroid patient. The major disadvantages, however, are that there is generally a delay in controlling the hyperthyroidism and a high incidence of hypothyroidism. The delay before clinical improvement occurs is variable and cannot be predicted. It is generally optimistic to expect biochemical and clinical control in less than two to three months, and this period may be much longer. The treatment dose of radioiodine should, therefore, be followed by a period on antithyroid drugs to achieve early clinical control. Some patients will require a second dose of radioiodine and a minimum period of one year should be allowed between doses.

The most important and frequent complication of radioiodine treatment is hypothyroidism, and 10–15% of patients develop this during the first year after treatment, and a further 3–6% became hypothyroid annually thereafter. The prevalence of hypothyroidism after 10 years lies at 40–60% and approaches 80% after 15 years. Many factors modify the biological effects of radioiodine and only some of these can be measured; thus it is not possible to calculate the "correct" dose for a patient.

Radioiodine is not an ideal treatment for hyperthyroidism, but is, nevertheless, the most satisfactory form of destructive treatment for some patients.

Management of the individual patient

Neonatal hyperthyroidism—This is an acute self-limiting condition that will remit in three to four months. Treatment should be with iodides and antithyroid drugs for this period, and the dose should be adjusted on clinical grounds. Exchange transfusion may be justified in the severely hyperthyroid neonate.

Hyperthyroidism in children—This generally occurs in the second decade. Antithyroid drug treatment should be used for one to three years, and if subsequent relapse occurs the patient should be treated surgically.

Hyperthyroidism in young adults—There are two recognised courses of action open to this age group. Firstly, the patient may be treated with antithyroid drugs (and thyroxine) for one to two years. The relapse rate is about 30% after one year and 45–55% after 10 years. Relapse should be treated surgically. The practice of giving patients repeated courses of antithyroid drugs is to be deprecated. Alternatively partial thyroidectomy may be performed as soon as the patient has been adequately controlled with antithyroid drugs and thyroxine. The advantage is that the hyperthyroidism is treated directly, the immunological status of the patient is altered, and the risk of severe ophthalmic problems is reduced. The disadvantage is that surgery is performed on about half the patients who will achieve long-term remission after a single course of antithyroid drugs. Patients in this age group, therefore, should be treated with antithyroid drugs and surgery should be reserved for a relapse. Surgery should be considered in the first episode in patients with severe disease, a large goitre, or an ophthalmopathy of any severity.

Hyperthyroidism in pregnancy—This should usually be controlled with antithyroid drugs together with thyroxine to prevent fetal hypothyroidism. The minimum effective dose of carbimazole should be used since this drug crosses the placenta and may cause goitre in the fetus. Breast-feeding must be avoided if it is necessary to continue treatment during the puerperium since the thionamide drugs are excreted in the milk.

Hyperthyroidism in middle-aged and elderly patients—These patients should normally be treated with radioiodine followed by antithyroid drugs after a week. Thyroxine should be added when the patient becomes euthyroid. Drugs should be discontinued after 12 months to reassess the patient's thyroid state and a further dose of radioiodine given if the patient remains hyperthyroid. Hyperthyroidism should be controlled with drugs before administering radioiodine in patients with major cardiovascular problems. It is, of course, necessary to discontinue the antithyroid drugs for one week before and one week after the dose. Subsequent control should follow the lines indicated above. A case can be made for intentional radioiodine ablation in hyperthyroidism.

Nodular goitre—Hyperthyroidism due to a nodular goitre should normally be treated surgically (after drug control) in the younger patient but may be treated by radioiodine in the older patient if pressure symptoms are not present.

Thyroid crisis—The management of crisis should include intravenous sodium iodide, oral carbimazole, propranolol, and parenteral steroids. Supportive treatment must provide intravenous fluids, oxygen administration to combat anoxia, and digoxin and diuretics if cardiac failure occurs.

EXTRATHYROIDAL MANIFESTATIONS OF GRAVES'S DISEASE

Ophthalmopathy—Minor degrees of ophthalmopathy do not need treatment. Ophthalmic problems are less troublesome if the patient is rendered permanently euthyroid early in the disease. (1) Discomfort and grittiness in the eyes may generally be relieved by methylcellulose eye drops. (2) Lid retraction may be distressing to patients and may be relieved in some by guanethidine eye drops. These do, however, have the disadvantage that they cause conjunctival irritation in many patients. (3) Proptosis and congestive ophthalmopathy: these should normally be managed by a specialist unit. Steroids and other immunosuppressives, tarsorrhaphy, orbital decompression, and orbital irradiation may all play a part in managing these problems.

Dermopathy—Minor degrees of localised myxoedema do not need treatment. More extensive lesions are best treated with local steroid preparations under occlusive polyethylene dressings. Areas that are resistant to this form of treatment will usually respond to local infiltration with triamcinolone.

HYPOTHYROIDISM

There is general agreement that all patients with symptomatic hypothyroidism should receive replacement treatment.

Management

Thyroxine should be used in the routine management of hypothyroidism. The initial dose should not exceed 0·05 mg daily in patients over 40; an initial dose of 0·1 mg daily may be used in younger patients. The dose should be increased by increments until the patient is clinically and biochemically euthyroid. The optimum dose varies between 0·1 and 0·2 mg daily and higher doses are rarely needed. There is no need for triiodothyronine or tablets combining thyroxine and triiodothyronine in routine management, since these confer no additional symptomatic benefit, side effects are more common, and serum triiodothyronine levels are normal on thyroxine as there is a substantial extrathyroidal conversion of thyroxine to triiodothyronine. A raised serum thyroxine concentration is not, therefore, an essential prerequisite for adequate replacement treatment as has been claimed. There is only one particular indication for the long-term maintenance of a patient on triiodothyronine in preference to thyroxine: in patients who have had total thyroid ablation for thyroid carcinoma, treatment should be stopped at regular intervals so that scanning procedures may be carried out. The replacement treatment may be discontinued for a considerably shorter time if triiodothyronine is used. It is important to ensure that adequate hormone is given to suppress thyroid-stimulating hormone secretion in these patients since this is a major part of their management.

Treatment of thyroid disease

Replacement treatment with thyroxine must be introduced cautiously in patients with ischaemic heart disease, in whom it may not be possible to give full replacement doses. The addition of a beta-adrenergic blocker such as propranolol, which can be increased incrementally with the thyroxine, may allow patients with angina pectoris to tolerate a larger dose of thyroxine than would otherwise be possible.

There is no general agreement on the best treatment for hypothyroid (myxoedema) coma. It is common practice to give thyroxine in doses of 0·05 mg daily by mouth combined with triiodothyronine 20–40 µg daily by intramuscular injection together with hydrocortisone hemisuccinate 100 mg twice daily. Supportive treatment with fluids, assisted respiration, and treatment for cardiac failure or arrhythmias should be provided. The body temperature should be slowly raised to normal. It must be remembered that over-enthusiastic therapeutic activity can be as dangerous as inactivity in patients with coma.

GOITRE

A goitre is an enlargement of the thyroid gland, and is common in the general population, even in areas where iodine deficiency is not endemic (10–15% of women and 1–3% of men). Physiological thyroid enlargement commonly occurs at puberty and during pregnancy. It is not possible to detect any disturbance of thyroid function or discover any aetiological factor in most patients, and no treatment is needed other than reassurance. Thyroid enlargement may not be associated with any disturbance of thyroid function and the management of those conditions that commonly present as goitre is as follows.

THYROIDITIS

Autoimmune thyroiditis

The term autoimmune thyroiditis defines the group of conditions characterised by the presence of circulating thyroid antibodies and sometimes of immunologically competent cells capable of reacting with some thyroid constituents. This group includes those conditions that have been classified as Hashimoto's disease, lymphadenoid goitre, and lymphocytic thyroiditis. There is no specific treatment for autoimmune thyroiditis. Replacement treatment with thyroxine (T4) should be started only in patients with symptomatic hypothyroidism and those euthyroid patients with a raised serum thyrotrophin (TSH) concentration and a goitre that is causing pressure symptoms or placing the patient at a cosmetic disadvantage. The objective of treatment is to relieve symptoms and reduce thyroid size. Sufficient T4 should be given to suppress pituitary TSH secretion. There is no justification for treating asymptomatic patients with T4 and such treatment will not slow the progression of the thyroiditis. Surgical reduction of goitre is rarely needed and should only be carried out if severe pressure symptoms are present.

Subacute (De Quervain's) thyroiditis

No treatment other than simple analgesics is needed in mild cases of subacute thyroiditis. Most doctors agree that steroids are most effective in controlling symptoms in the more severe cases. The clinical response is rapid, and the initial high dose of steroid (30–40 mg prednisone or equivalent a day) can be rapidly reduced and discontinued after two to four weeks in most patients. It is alleged that relapses are more frequent if steroids are used but this probably only reflects their use in the more severe cases. It is also claimed that the addition of T4 or triiodothyronine (T3) may suppress pituitary TSH secretion, but this lacks proof and seems inherently unlikely since TSH will be suppressed by the rapid discharge of preformed hormone in the acute stages. Sulphonamides, antibiotics, iodine, antithyroid drugs, and irradiation have all been used. There is nothing to recommend any of them, and irradiation almost certainly increases the risk of subsequent hypothyroidism.

The acute stage of the disease may be complicated by transient hyperthyroidism but this does not require treatment. Treatment would in any event present problems since the hyperthyroidism results from the discharge of previously synthesised hormone from the gland. Hypothyroidism if it occurs is treated with T4 (see above).

Invasive fibrous (Riedel's) thyroiditis

The treatment of Riedel's thyroiditis is primarily directed towards relieving pressure symptoms and most patients need partial thyroidectomy. The disease may become static later or may recur producing further pressure symptoms. No pharmacological preparation is of any value. Thyroid failure may occur if the disease is extensive and should be treated with T4 (see above).

TUMOURS OF THE THYROID

Most thyroid tumours arise from the epithelial elements of the gland, and neoplasms of mesenchymal origin are uncommon. The gross and histological features of both benign and malignant thyroid tumours show wide variations. Many classifications have tended to emphasise these differences, but there is little clinical or therapeutic justification for an elaborate taxonomy.

Tumours of follicular cell origin

Adenoma—The major clinical importance of the thyroid adenoma lies in the need to distinguish between this lesion and carcinoma. The correct surgical procedure is excision biopsy.

Treatment of thyroid disease

Papillary and follicular carcinoma—There is no absolute agreement on the correct treatment of differentiated thyroid carcinoma. Total thyroidectomy should probably be carried out in all patients since at least 60% of these tumours can be shown to be multicentric. Good results may be obtained by hemithyroidectomy in some patients but small foci of carcinoma in the other lobe are often invisible to the naked eye, and this procedure cannot be generally recommended (and is associated with a considerably reduced survival time). The major complications of total thyroidectomy are damage to the external laryngeal nerves, recurrent laryngeal nerve injury, and hypoparathyroidism. The patient should then be started on replacement treatment with T4 or T3 if no secondary deposits are present. The treatment should restore euthyroidism and suppress pituitary TSH secretion. The TSH level must be suppressed since many well-differentiated tumours are dependent on TSH.

If present, cervical node metastases are generally mobile and should be excised. The patient with lymph node metastases should be left without replacement treatment for the first two months. The patient should become hypothyroid during this time and endogenous TSH levels will rise. A high-dose (200–500 μCi) ^{131}I scan should be carried out after further stimulation with exogenous TSH (10 units intramuscularly). If there are any areas of localised uptake of ^{131}I the patient should be given a therapeutic dose of 100–150 mCi of radioiodine. One week after treatment or immediately after the scan if no functional tissue has been shown the patient should start replacement treatment with T3 in sufficient quantities (60 mcg/day) to suppress TSH secretion. Treatment should be stopped annually or earlier if there is clinical or radiological evidence of recurrence and a further scan (200–500 μCi) carried out. A further large dose of ^{131}I may be given before restarting replacement treatment. The advantage of T3 is that it has a shorter half-life than T4 and the patient is, therefore, subjected to the symptoms of hypothyroidism for a shorter period each year.

The management of the patient with skeletal or pulmonary metastases should follow similar lines. Thyroidectomy should be followed by radioiodine treatment (100–150 mCi) after about two months. The patient should subsequently receive replacement treatment with T3, but it may be desirable to give the patient further therapeutic doses of ^{131}I at intervals of a few weeks to a few months in the early stages of treatment. (^{131}I scans in patients with distant metastases should be done using at least 1mCi.) No rigid schedule can be specified for patients in the early stages and T3 should be stopped and a scan performed, with subsequent treatment if indicated, on the basis of regular clinical and radiological assessment. Annual assessment may be instituted when ^{131}I uptake has been reduced to negligible proportions and no residual tumour can be detected radiologically or clinically. There are few major problems associated with ^{131}I treatment, and the number of cases of leukaemia reported is only just into double figures. The overall five-year survival rate for well-differentiated carcinoma is 75–80%.

Anaplastic and other poorly differentiated tumours—Surgery has little to offer in the management of these tumours, which infiltrate widely and rapidly into adjacent tissues. Many anaplastic tumours are relatively radioinsensitive, and the major objective of external beam irradiation is palliation. Reduction in tumour mass, the prevention of obstruction, ulceration, or haemorrhage will all help to make the patient's terminal phase more comfortable. The overall five-year survival rate is less than 20%. Radioiodine plays no part in the management of the undifferentiated tumour.

Tumours of parafollicular cell origin

Most medullary carcinomata are slow growing, and surgery offers the best chance of cure. Total thyroidectomy should be carried out since many of these tumours are multifocal in origin. Lymph node metastases should also be excised if possible. Partial resection should be attempted if the complete neoplasm cannot be removed since this may lead to partial relief of symptoms. External beam irradiation should be applied if it is not possible to resect the tumour fully, although this is not always effective. The treatment's success and patient's progress should be monitored by serial measurements of the calcitonin levels. The patient must be given replacement doses of T_4 after ablative treatment. The mean survival time from diagnosis is about five years.

The management of coincidental hyperparathyroidism or phaeochromocytoma should follow standard lines. Diarrhoea may be troublesome and does not always respond to standard remedies. Therapeutic successes with indomethacin and nutmeg have been reported recently.

Tumours of mesodermal and mixed origin

Lymphoma—Treatment for lymphoma of the thyroid should be by external beam irradiation. Thyroidectomy is carried out in some patients before the diagnosis is made histologically. Surgery should always be followed by external beam treatment. Replacement treatment with T_4 will be required by most patients. The five-year survival rate is about 20%.

Teratoma—This is rare. It is almost invariably benign in childhood but is generally malignant if detected in adult life (presumably the result of malignant change in a small and previously undetected teratoma). Surgery is the only treatment available.

Other tumours—Fibrosarcoma, mixed osteogenic and chondrogenic tumours, and the extremely rare haemangioendothelioma of the thyroid are all highly malignant and not generally amenable to treatment.

Endemic goitre

Endemic goitre and endemic cretinism rank among the world's most common major health problems. The role of iodine deficiency in causing endemic goitre is unquestioned, although local factors (such as ingested goitrogens) may play a contributory part in some areas. Treatment of affected communities may be achieved by iodisation of water or salt or by the injection of iodised oil, which provides a depot of iodine that is sufficient for several years. These methods are cheap and simple to apply and thus the problems of endemic goitre and endemic cretinism are potentially eradicable.

Dyshormonogenetic goitre

Dyshormonogenetic goitre is rare. Patients invariably have a goitre (which is TSH-dependent) but do not always show the clinical features of hypothyroidism. Treatment should be with T_4 in sufficient doses to suppress pituitary TSH secretion. There will be a substantial reduction in the size of the goitre unless irreversible degenerative changes have occurred in the gland. Treatment must be started as soon as the diagnosis is made in the infant or child to prevent permanent impairment of cerebral function or retardation of bone growth.

Modern approach to diabetes mellitus

J M STOWERS

Diabetes may be functionally defined as a relative or absolute deficiency of insulin that may or may not be associated with symptoms. There are several different reasons for insulin insufficiency but the net result is the syndrome of diabetes. It is important to recognise the many years that usually elapse between the appearance of the first stigmata or chemical abnormality of diabetes and the presentation of the patient because of the primary symptoms, for the chronic mild hyperglycaemia and hyperlipidaemia are significantly correlated with ischaemic heart disease, atheroma more generally, and with retinopathy and precocious development of cataracts. About 20% of new diabetics presenting to clinics already have recognisable diabetic complications. If diabetes is diagnosed early, perhaps as a result of investigating symptomless glycosuria or because of recognising a characteristic known to correlate with diabetes, it is certain that simple treatment can delay the onset of such degenerative complications, which are likely to disable a patient far more than the mere presence of mild diabetes itself. Diabetes is the commonest endocrine disease in Britain, affecting overtly at least 2% of the population, and thus the epidemiological approach assumes major importance, since it should facilitate early recognition, explanation to the patient, and his co-operation in effective treatment.

The general practitioner is best placed to find the people at risk and arrange for them to be screened for diabetes. The criteria for screening are: strong family history of diabetes in first-degree relatives; symptomless glycosuria; chronic obesity; and precocious onset of occlusive arterial disease, especially in women before the menopause. The obstetric data are: multiparity (more than four pregnancies lasting at least 28 weeks); heavy-for-dates baby, remembering maternal height and gestational age—for example, over 4·5 kg for a woman of average height after 40 weeks gestation; glycosuria to Clinistix in a second fasting urine specimen; one or more stillbirths or neonatal deaths; islet hyperplasia in pancreas of stillborn baby in absence of Rh isoimmunisation; congenital anomaly in baby; hydramnios; and history of two or more abortions.

If chemical diabetes—that is, abnormal glucose tolerance but a normal fasting blood sugar level—is confirmed by oral or intravenous glucose tolerance tests, dietary treatment is usually sufficient to restore glucose tolerance to normal. Such treatment includes reduction of excess weight in the obese and restriction of refined carbohydrate in those of normal weight. If these measures prove inadequate small doses of sulphonylureas can apparently often reverse chemical diabetes in patients aged 35 or under. By the time overt diabetes has developed in a patient with a normal weight and without intercurrent illness the possibility of reversing diabetes is extremely remote.

OVERT DIABETES

Patients with mild overt diabetes with fasting capillary blood sugar levels from 6·7 mmol/l (120 mg/100 ml) to 11·1 mmol/l (200 mg/100 ml) may usually be treated by diet alone if there is associated obesity, but not so predictably if the patient is of normal weight or thin. While the energy content of the diet has to be tailored to the degree the patient is overweight, other features are more consistent. Thus refined carbohydrate, which would call for a greater insulin response than the patient can achieve, should be omitted in food taken in smallish meals. In this way hyperglycaemic peaks may be avoided, for the blood sugar level is still the best measure of the degree of control. Generally this means taking food in as natural a state as possible—that is, when it is more bulky to satisfy the appetite of the naturally hungry yet only slowly converted into its constituent sugars, amino-acids, and fatty acids.

Other qualitative aspects of food selection are more controversial, but as, for ethical reasons, hard biological facts are difficult to obtain in man, it seems rational to rely on more definite animal studies and on the weight of circumstantial human evidence. Thus epidemiologists have shown clearly a close association between a plasma cholesterol level above about 5·2 mmol/l (210 mg/100 ml) plasma and a rise in the mortality from ischaemic heart disease. Diabetes is associated with a tendency to hypercholesterolaemia because of relative insufficiency of insulin and to some extent because of the relatively high proportion of fat to carbohydrate in most diabetic diets not designed for weight reduction. About two-thirds of the body cholesterol pool is synthesised and the remaining one-third is derived from saturated animal fat in the diet, largely egg yolk and dairy products. Unsaturated fats, mainly vegetable fats, can actually lower the plasma cholesterol level more than a fat-free diet. These considerations suggest that replacing as much saturated fat by unsaturated fat as possible by suitable selection of commonly available foods would tend to reduce atherosclerosis in diabetics in parallel with the long-term fall in the serum cholesterol level. This is not a fact but circumstantial evidence makes it highly probable, and where the stakes are high such leads are worth following.

TABLETS

The advent of treating diabetics with tablets on a large scale opened a new era, the full implications of which are now becoming apparent. The sulphonylureas enabled many patients with maturity onset diabetes without ketonuria to control their blood sugar when diet alone was insufficient and when insulin was the only alternative. The bright prospects of tablet treatment have recently been marred by reports of increased cardiovascular mortality in patients taking the sulphonylurea, tolbutamide, to be followed a little later by even worse results with the biguanide, phenformin, compared with patients treated by diet alone or diet and insulin.

Evidence is by no means one-sided but there seems to be little doubt that sulphonylurea drugs are associated with an increased mortality rate after myocardial infarction. Such considerations must temper our approach to the treatment of long-term diabetes, and more and better trials are needed to compare the cardiovascular risks of treatment with insulin and with sulphonylureas.

Sulphonylureas

The number of commercially available sulphonylureas continues to proliferate, more for commercial than medical reasons for there is little to choose between the properties of the last three additions to the list —glibenclamide, glipizide, and glibornuride. They are suitable when diet alone has proved inadequate and in diabetics without ketonuria, but they are not the best treatment for the maturity onset diabetic who is still notably obese. Nevertheless, sulphonylureas may sometimes usefully supplement the hypoglycaemic action of biguanides that have been used initially in treating obese maturity-onset diabetics.

All the sulphonylureas may produce rashes in about 3% of patients, and there is some cross-reactivity between the different drugs. When this occurs it is worth trying glymidine (Gondafon) as it is chemically most distinct being actually a sulphapyrimidine, rather than a sulphonylurea. Flushing after alcohol occurs with several of these drugs but most consistently with chlorpropamide, which also has a definite but rare association with cholestatic jaundice. Dyspeptic side effects, however, are more likely to occur with the shorter-acting compounds that are usually given more than once a day before meals.

Hypoglycaemia is an overdose effect rather than a side effect but has been troublesome, mainly when there has been a failure to recognise the great potency of small doses of compounds such as glibenclamide or glipizide: as little as 2·5 mg may cause hypoglycaemic coma. It is important to remember the long biological half life (about 40 hours) of chlorpropamide, for in the presence of renal failure even a small daily dose may lead to an excess accumulating in the plasma, so that long-lasting hypoglycaemia may occur, particularly in elderly diabetics living alone. This type of hypoglycaemia is harder to treat than the more transient type due to insulin overdose, not only because of the long persistence of the chlorpropamide in the blood but because it inhibits

TABLE I—*Sulphonylureas: comparative features*

Official name	Proprietary name	Tablet size (mg)	Range of dose (mg)	Potency	Approximate biological half life (h)	Particular aspects
Acetohexamide	Dimelor	500	500–1500	Medium	5	
Chlorpropamide	Diabinese Melitase	100 250	100–500	Strong	40	Flushing after alcohol, occasional cholestatic jaundice
Glibenclamide	Daonil Euglucon	5	2·5–25	Strong and quick	12	
Glibornuride	Glutril	25	12·5–75	Strong	8	
Glipizide	Glibenese Minidiab	5	2·5–30	Strong	3·5	
Glymidine	Gondafon	500	500–2000	Medium	4	A sulphapyrimidine with virtually no cross-reaction with sulphonylureas in regard to rashes
Tolazamide	Tolanase	100 250	100–750	Strong	7	
Tolbutamide	Promidex Rastinon	500	500–3000	Relatively weak	4	Metabolite gives flakey precipitate with sulphosalicylic acid or picric acid (Esbach's reagent) or when acidified and boiled; hence false-positive tests for proteinuria (not with Albustix)

TABLE II—*Biguanides: comparative features*

Official name	Proprietary name	Tablet size (mg)	Range of dose (mg)	Particular aspects
Metformin	Glucophage Metiguanide	500, 850	500–3000	
Phenformin	Dibotin Dibotin SA Dipar SR Meltrol SR	25 50 50 50	25–300	Occasional severe lactic acidosis, especially with renal or hepatic failure, ischaemia, or after alcohol

the glucose-6-phosphatase in the liver needed for the release of glucose from glycogen. Injected glucagon may then prove effective and glucose needs to be given by continuous infusion over many hours and not just as a single intravenous dose as is the case after an overdose of short-acting insulins. Table I gives comparative features of the sulphonylurea drugs now available in Britain.

Biguanides

The biguanides have done much to improve the oral treatment of diabetic patients who have the dual problem of continuing obesity and hyperglycaemia without ketonuria, for in carefully adjusted doses they may favour loss of weight without risk of hypoglycaemia. Patients may continue to have high blood sugar levels in spite of calorie restriction or may simply have failed to restrict their diet properly after adequate instruction. Left with the choice of letting them suffer the inevitable consequences of precocious cataract, neuropathy, and atheroma that follow chronic hyperglycaemia it is rational to build up the dose of the biguanide slowly to a point where the appetite and the weight begin to fall. Metabolic studies have shown that the weight so lost is due not only to eating less but also to actual malabsorption, which may occur for essential elements such as folic acid and vitamin B_{12} as well as for the diet more generally. Patients on more than about 2 g metformin a day should be screened about once a year for low levels of plasma folate and B_{12}. These will rise on withdrawing metformin or alternatively folic acid and B_{12} may be used as supplements to the diet.

Phenformin in large doses has purposely been omitted from this account, for there is a definite if small risk of lactic acidosis developing in a few diabetics taking over about 100 mg/day—even if they have no evidence of renal or hepatic failure or known ischaemic disease, which are positive contraindications to its use. The fact that, unlike metformin, phenformin is concentrated in the liver may help to explain its greater association with clinical lactic acidosis, for the liver is normally a main site of lactate uptake. The biguanides are often used to control the blood sugar level after a secondary failure of a sulphonylurea, the two types of drug having quite different mechanisms. The biguanides increase the permeability of cells in general to glucose but do not increase endogenous insulin production. Occasionally it is worth introducing a biguanide in modest doses to insulin-dependent diabetics to reduce their tendency to unpredictable hypoglycaemic attacks. The biguanide may partly replace insulin by a drug which in itself causes no risk of hypoglycaemia. This is seldom necessary if insulin is used intelligently by the patient and his adviser.

The therapeutic dose of biguanides is often near to the dose that will start to produce side effects, which occur in the following order:

anorexia, nausea, and then vomiting or diarrhoea, or both, with associated malaise. Susceptibility to such side effects varies greatly between individuals, and they occur more often if the dosage of the drug is increased too quickly. Withdrawal of the biguanide produces an improvement within eight hours. Rashes are less often associated with the biguanides than with the sulphonylureas.

The biguanides are no better than sulphonylureas in relation to long-term vascular effects. In the University Group Diabetes Programme study, in which phenformin was used in a dose of 100 mg/day, the cardiovascular mortality was over two and a half times that in the diet-treated group, despite the fact that phenformin's potential to lower cholesterol and triglyceride levels in the plasma and produce fibrinolysis might have been expected to exert a favourable effect. The comparative features of the two biguanides are given in table II.

INSULIN

The aim in treating diabetes is to achieve biochemical normality, and the most relevant single test is still measurement of the blood sugar level. In the non-diabetic the level of plasma insulin varies in relation to the intake of carbohydrate and protein, so that the diurnal fluctuation in blood sugar may stay within a range of about 1·7 mmol/l (30 mg/100 ml). If diabetics are studied on regular identical feeds every two hours during the day before they start insulin treatment the blood sugar will usually tend to be considerably higher in the late morning than in the evening, presumably representing the net effect of hormones that tend to antagonise the small amount of residual insulin they produce. Such a diabetic needs treatment with an insulin that acts most strongly in the morning, but it will certainly be impracticable to achieve the narrow limits of normal blood sugar control seen in the non-diabetic without risking potentially dangerous hypoglycaemia. We have not yet achieved the necessary fine adjustment of insulin administration except by complicated computerised artificial pancreas machines that can continuously monitor the blood sugar and infuse insulin as needed to achieve a predetermined level of glycaemia.

Although new insulins are still being introduced, old ones are seldom withdrawn, so that we now have available 17 different kinds, each one in at least two different strengths. These are classified in the table.

It is most important for doctors to know well a useful range of insulins rather than spread their experience too thinly. There are theoretical and some practical advantages in avoiding the addition of proteins to insulin for they increase the incidence of local skin reactions and antibody formation. Similarly, neutral rather than acid insulins produce less subcutaneous fat atrophy. Finally, porcine insulin is less

TABLE III—*Insulins: Comparative table*

Standard preparations	Strengths μ/ml	Duration of action	Peak(s) of action (h)	pH	Appearance	Source	Added protein	Special features
Soluble:								
Unmodified	20, 40, 80, 320	Short	2–5	Acid	Clear	Mainly beef	o	
Neutral	40, 80	Short	2–5	Neutral	Clear	Mainly beef	o	
Zinc suspension lente 30% SL .. .. 70% UL	40, 80	Intermediate–long	3–6 and 6–12	Neutral	Cloudy	30% pig 70% beef	o	
Zinc suspension semilente	40, 80	Intermediate	3–6	Neutral	Cloudy	Pig	o	
Zinc suspension ultralente	40, 80	Long	6–12	Neutral	Cloudy	Beef	o	
Isophane	40, 80	Intermediate	3–6	Neutral	Cloudy	Beef	+	Contains no excess of protamine and zinc uncombined with insulin
Protamine zinc ..	40, 80	Long	5–14	Neutral	Cloudy	Beef	+	Contains excess of protamine and zinc uncombined with insulin
Globin zinc	80	Intermediate	3–5	Neutral	Clear	Beef	+	
Highly purified:								
Neutral								
Actrapid MC ..	40, 80	Short	2–5	Neutral	Clear	Pig	o	Virtually non-antigenic
Leo neutral ..	40, 80	Short	2–5	Neutral	Clear	Pig	o	Wise to reduce by about 20% when first changing from less pure insulin in amounts greater than about 40 units a day

TABLE III—*Insulins: Comparative table*

Standard preparations	Strengths u/ml	Duration of action	Peak(s) of action (h)	pH	Appearance	Source	Added protein	Special features
Highly purified—cont.								
Semilente type Semitard MC	40, 80	Intermediate	3–6	Neutral	Cloudy	Pig	0	,,
Lente type .. Monotard MC	40, 80	Intermediate–long	3–12	Neutral	Cloudy	Pig	0	,,
Isophane .. Leo Retard ..	40, 80	Intermediate	3–6	Neutral	Cloudy	Pig	0	
Proinsulin-freed:								
Zinc suspension lente Lentard .. 30% SL .. 70% UL ..	40, 80	Intermediate–long	3–6 and 6–12	Neutral	Cloudy	30% pig 70% beef	0	Less antigenic than standard preparations but more antigenic than highly purified pig insulins
Zinc suspension semilente ..	40–80	Intermediate	3–6	Neutral	Cloudy	Pig	0	,,
Zinc suspension ultralente Ultratard ..	40–80	Long	6–12	Neutral	Cloudy	Beef	0	,,
Biphasic .. Rapitard ..	40–80	Intermediate–long	2–5 and 6–13	Neutral	Cloudy	25% pork 75% beef	0	,,

Since insulin preparations of similar name are now marketed in three grades of purification and vary in their antigenicity the name of the specific preparation should be prescribed in full.

antigenic in man than bovine, but there is not enough porcine insulin to satisfy the world demand.

Apart from the animal source of insulin its purity is important in determining its antigenicity. The impurity of biggest molecular size is proinsulin, and the Novo Company has now marketed four insulins, some pork and some beef, from which virtually all proinsulin has been removed. When porcine insulin is highly purified the least antigenic insulin preparations are produced. So far such insulins are marketed by only two companies, both Danish. They are available in short, intermediate, and long-acting forms, but the short-acting tends to be rather shorter in duration than the more antigenic standard soluble insulin, and the long-acting Monotard tends to be of rather shorter duration than the standard ultralente preparation, because porcine insulin zinc suspension does not form crystals as well as the beef variety.

Antibodies to insulin normally form within three months of starting treatment, and at high levels they delay the hypoglycaemic agent of the insulin. Monocomponent or Leo neutral insulins do not do this, but perhaps the best reasons for using these highly purified porcine preparations at present are for the occasional insulin-resistant patient, patients with local fat dystrophy, and possibly also for pregnant diabetics. The zones of fat hypertrophy do not seem to occur at the sites of injections of these insulins, and zones of fat atrophy may be made to fill in when they are injected peripherally into the atrophic areas.

An important feature of these highly purified insulins is that a 10–20% smaller dose may be needed compared with that of the standard types or even that of the less purified pig insulins. This reduced need may become apparent right away or over weeks or months as the level of insulin antibodies declines. If a change to monocomponent or Leo neutral is to be made because of resistance to a standard insulin, it is wise to undertake the change under close surveyance and to reduce the dose as an initial trial by 20% before making further adjustments according to the results obtained. Less difficulty with overdose effects is likely when 40 units a day or less of standard insulin is needed.

Most young diabetics can be better controlled on two daily doses of a short-acting insulin than on a single daily dose of a longer-acting one. As they should have a long life expectancy, it seems to be worth their while to take this amount of extra trouble to avoid or at least postpone the disabling long-term complications of the disease. When starting a diabetic on a two-dose insulin regimen it is helpful to divide the previous daily dose into thirds and to give just under two-thirds before breakfast and just under one-third before the main evening meal. If the patient does hard physical work in the day the proportion of insulin given before breakfast should be reduced. The total dose of the twice-daily insulin is slightly reduced at first to avoid heralding the new regimen with hypoglycaemia, which may discredit it in the patient's eyes. The morning and evening doses or scales of doses may then be cautiously adjusted to achieve optimal control.

Success in this, as in other aspects of insulin treatment, will only be achieved by the well-informed co-operation of the patient: thus adequate written and verbal instruction of all diabetics newly starting insulin is one of the most important goals of treatment. Their instruction should include information on how to regulate their dose according to Clinitests done mainly before breakfast and before the evening meal. The result of the morning test is used to regulate the evening dose which controls it and for the same reason the evening test is used to regulate the morning dose. Basing the morning and evening doses on the urine tests done at these same times is irrational and likely to lead to unnecessary wide fluctuations of blood sugar.

Single daily dosage

Older patients on usually smaller doses of insulin may be able to achieve satisfactory regulation on a single daily dose. This should be regulated by a Clinitest done on freshly formed urine passed when the insulin is expected to be maximally active, for in this way it is relatively safe for the patient to increase the dose to improve poor test results without risking hypoglycaemia at other times of the day or night. Even mild hypoglycaemia may lead to subsequent reactive hyperglycaemia lasting for a day or so. Thus hyperglycaemia is usually an indication to increase the dose of insulin if there has been no hypoglycaemic episode in the previous 24 hours. If, on the other hand, the hyperglycaemia has followed previous hypoglycaemia it is an indication to reduce the dose of insulin which precipitated it. In this way the peaks and troughs of blood sugar may be decreased on a smaller total daily dose of insulin. Such reactive hyperglycaemia is reduced in patients on full doses of beta-blocking drugs, which therefore leave insulin-dependent diabetics at a normally unjustifiably greater risk of developing severe hypoglycaemia without the usual warning signs.

Diabetes is perhaps the best example of a chronic disease where the full instruction of the patient and his willing co-operation are the prime factors in his present and future well-being.

Obesity

J F MUNRO

The medical management of obesity is notoriously unsatisfactory. Only a relatively small percentage of patients lose weight effectively, and a large proportion of these subsequently regain weight.[1] Weight loss, however, is only one aspect of managing the overweight patient, who will have sought medical advice either because of obesity or for some other reason that may or may not be a complication of obesity. The finding of a condition such as diabetes, ischaemic heart disease, or a hiatus hernia may provide a clear-cut justification for recommending weight loss. Sometimes, however, emphasis on weight loss may be unrealistic and of secondary importance when compared with other aspects of their management, such as stopping smoking in the obese, breathless, chronic bronchitic.

Patients who seek medical advice primarily for obesity are often distressed for cultural or psychological, rather than physical, reasons. They are a self-selected group who have failed with self-imposed dietary control and often with other measures, which may have included membership of one of the various slimming clubs (these latter produce satisfactory results for many patients).[2] This self-selection may possibly explain in part why results obtained in clinical practice are often disappointing. If the doctor is to help he must first try to determine the reason for the request for medical help. Patients will only reduce if they are appropriately motivated and are aware of the underlying cause of their weight gain. The direct question, 'Why do you want to lose weight?' will often provide a revealing answer. Sometimes it will show that the management should be primarily supportive as in those who have failed to appreciate that weight gain was caused by, rather than the cause of, some underlying unhappiness.

Many patients have an unrealistic concept of the expected rate of weight loss and are in danger of becoming disheartened while actually making satisfactory progress. To prevent this the clinician should explain that any initial dramatic reduction is largely caused by loss of fluid, rather than fat, cannot be maintained, and may indeed be followed by weight regain due to fluid retention. He should emphasise that an average weekly weight loss of "only" 0·5 kg is excellent and would result in an annual loss of 26 kg (almost exactly 4 stone). The patient must realise that factors other than degree of adiposity can affect weight in the short term and must be advised against weighing at intervals of less than one week and of paying excessive attention to weight change from week to week. The patient should be given the opportunity of attending at self-determined time intervals. Failure to make satisfactory progress should not provoke criticism, but rather further inquiry into the difficulties being experienced. In summary the doctor whose support has been sought must first achieve satisfactory rapport so that he can help the patient overcome various metabolic and psychological factors that tend to perpetuate obesity.

EXERCISE

In the absence of an effective thermogenic agent, increase in physical activity is the only method of increasing energy expenditure, which is characteristically less in the obese than the non-obese. Although considerable activity is required to utilise 1 kg of adipose tissue the need to encourage the obese to take exercise is absolute. It should be emphasised that walking an additional 1–2 miles daily should produce an annual loss of up to 6 kg provided that calorie consumption is kept constant. Unless there is a medical contraindication all obese patients should be given clear individual advice about the best way of increasing physical activity.

DIETARY CONTROL

The mainstay of any weight-reducing plan must be diet. Although many factors, including meal frequency and composition, may be of minor importance, the success of dietary control depends on the ability of the patient to adhere to a regimen that must provide fewer calories than the daily energy expenditure and lead to a permanent change in eating habits.

Sometimes a dietary history will show that both objectives may be achieved by permanently cutting out one or two items such as potatoes, sugar, or alcohol. More often, however, additional advice will be needed. Most obese people gain weight because of excessive carbohydrate consumption, and this emphasises the popularity of regimens based on carbohydrate rather than total calorie restriction. A calorie, however, is a calorie, and the regimen best suited to any one patient must take into account such considerations as occupation and may be found only by trial and error. Inadvertent cheating may most easily be detected, and corrected, by asking the patient to record accurately each total daily intake. Such a record may also show major faults in eating habit, such as nibbling while watching television or periods of uncontrollable carbohydrate gorging. It provides the basis of the behavioural approach, whereby the patient is first made aware of the various faults in his eating pattern by detailed recording of not only the nature and calorie value of food eaten, but also such aspects as time taken for meals, the place of eating, the degree of hunger and mood, physical position, and associated activities at time of eating. Corrective measures may then be introduced step by step and tailored to deal with the various faults. This approach is time consuming but may sometimes prove very effective.[3]

There are many commercially available low-calorie foods. These include formula diets such as Metercal and Slender, products such as Trimmets, Limmits, and Bisks, and various low-calorie soft drinks and crispbreads. Patients incapable of adhering to more conventional diets may achieve weight loss by substituting one or more meals with a "formula diet," but sooner or later they default from strict adherence and tend to regain weight. There is no evidence that the use of formula diets helps to correct basic faults in eating behaviour but low-calorie foods are of value if they can be incorporated on a permanent basis—for example low-calorie crispbreads may be substituted for bread and artificial sweeteners for sugar.

STARVATION

Although the dangers of therapeutic starvation have been reduced by a clearer understanding of the metabolic consequences of fasting, it is not without risk. The serious complications include electrolyte imbalances, cardiac arrhythmias, and, occasionally, sudden death. These hazards are such that costly stays in hospital are necessary. Therapeutic starvation, therefore, may only be justified if it produces long-term weight losses greater than those achieved by more conventional treatment. A critical appraisal of follow-up results after fasting for periods of up to three weeks show that this is not the case—either in patient with "refractory obesity" or at the time of initial referral to a hospital clinic.[4] The follow-up results remain disappointing even when therapeutic starvation is continued to within a few kilograms of ideal weight. In spite of correcting the metabolic consequences of obesity and despite the psychological incentives that might be expected from reduction to a personally and socially acceptable weight, rapid weight regain is common. It is difficult to justify prolonged fasting at least until some improved selection method can reduce the present high failure rate. It is important, however, to remember that weight change is only one aspect in managing obesity, and some patients may obtain tangible benefits from starvation despite subsequent regain in weight.

A low-calorie formula diet providing 0·75–1·5 MJ/day (180–360 kcal/day) has been suggested as an alternative to complete fasting and has the advantage that it can be used for outpatients. The regimen shares, however, the disadvantages of formula diets and its long-term efficacy is unestablished in patients who successfully adhere to it.

DRUGS

The value of the various drugs which have been used in managing obesity have recently been reviewed.[5] They can be assessed in terms of efficacy, side effects, and cost.

Obesity

Methylcellulose and other bulk agents are cheap, safe, and completely ineffective.

Biguanides produce modest weight reductions in non-diabetic subjects. Their mode of action is uncertain and their clinical value limited.

Thyroxine and triiodothyronine may produce weight loss in non-endocrine obesity, but their use is potentially hazardous and should be confined to patients with biochemical hypothyroidism.

Phenylethylamine derivatives

Phenylethylamine derivatives fall into three groups.

Amphetamine, D-amphetamine, and phenmetrazine are potential central nervous system (CNS) stimulants with anorectic properties and have been extensively abused. These drugs, and preparations containing them, should never be prescribed.

Phentermine, chlorphentermine, and diethylpropion are also CNS stimulants, but provided appropriate precautions are taken the danger of dependence appears to be acceptably low. When administered to patients with "refractory obesity" weight loss is disappointing and short-lived, and weight regain usually occurs when the drug is discontinued. Improved results may be obtained by earlier prescription but there is no firm evidence that the use of these, or any other drugs, facilitate a permanent change in eating habit. They should not be prescribed to patients with cardiovascular disease or hypertension. They are probably most effective in the depressed. They should be administered intermittently with intervals of not less than four weeks between monthly courses as this is as effective as, cheaper than, and less likely to cause addiction than continuous treatment. It should be explained to the patient that courses will only be repeated if significant weight regain does not occur during the four-week intervals, which should encourage the patient to establish good eating habit. Of the proprietary preparations of phentermine and diethylpropion available, Ionamin and Duromine are comparable while Apisate is cheaper than Dospan though both are paradoxically cheaper than Tenuate.

Fenfluramine, although structurally related to amphetamine, has anorectic properties without causing CNS stimulation. Drug dependence may develop but addiction is not a problem. Side effects include lethargy, diarrhoea and other gastrointestinal upsets, vivid dreams, and reversible alopecia, but the major drawback is depression, which is especially likely to occur if the drug is withdrawn abruptly.[6] For this reason it should never be prescribed intermittently and should be discontinued stepwise under close medical supervision. Given continuously, its anorectic effect is similar to that of intermittent phentermine but appears to last longer than the other amphetamine analogues and may be related to dosage. Individual response, however, is extremely variable. It is probably most effective in anxious, tense patients and should be avoided in the depressed. The theoretical advantage of Ponderax Pacaps (twice as distinct from thrice daily) does not justify the additional cost (table I).

Mazindol

Mazindol, although unrelated to the amphetamines, is a CNS stimulant. Some reports of its clinical efficacy are encouraging[7] but others are equally disappointing[8]; its major interest may be its chemical novelty.

TABLE *Cost of currently available anorectic drugs*

Approved name	Dose in mg	Proprietary name	Cost per 30 days at recommended dose*
Diethylpropion	75	Apisate	47p
	75	Tenuate Dospan	58p
	25	Tenuate	81p
Phentermine	30	Duromine	£1·35
		Ionamin	£1·26
Fenfluramine	120 tablets	Ponderax	£5·85
	120 capsules	Ponderax Pacaps	£6·49
Mazindol	2	Teronac	£3·13
L- & D-amphetamine	20	Durophet	70p
Phenmetrazine	30	Filon	£2·05
Phenbutrazate	20		

* Derived from *MIMS*, January, 1977.

BYPASS SURGERY

During the past few years an increasing number of patients with morbid obesity have undergone various bypass operations designed to produce weight loss by inducing a state of malabsorption. The most popular procedure is an end-to-side anastomosis of the first 33 cm of jejunum with the terminal 10 cm of ileum. The immediate operative mortality is about 4%. The operation results in steatorrhoea and explosive diarrhoea is common. This may be associated with excessive and distressing flatulence, anal excoriation, and prolapsing haemorrhoids, though these symptoms may settle with time. Other complications include an increase in the formation of renal and gall stones and impairment of liver function, occasionally resulting in hepatic failure. Polyarthritis is not uncommon; electrolyte imbalances are the rule; and without appropriate replacement treatment vitamin deficiencies may occur. Life-long medical follow-up is essential as the long-term consequences have yet to be evaluated. There is some evidence to suggest that the complications may be reduced by end-to-end anastomosis and by leaving a longer segment of ileum in continuity.

After the operation patients occasionally fail to lose weight. Others may reduce to less than their ideal weight and require re-anastomosis. Most, however, lose some 30–40 kg and then their weight stabilises within two years of surgery while still considerably above the ideal.[9] Most express themselves satisfied with the operation and many benefit psychologically.[10] The immediate mortality, postoperative complications, and uncertainty about the long-term effects, however, are such that bypass surgery should only be undertaken as a last resort in patients with gross morbid obesity and in centres where its ultimate efficacy can be objectively evaluated.

CONCLUSIONS

For weight loss to be effective it must be sustained. This can be achieved by bypass surgery, a multilative operation with an appreciable mortality, inevitable side effects, and unknown long-term sequelae. The alternatives to surgery are to promote energy expenditure by considerably increasing daily physical activity or permanently to alter previous bad eating habit by making appropriate changes in diet. Some patients fail to achieve this change, and there is very little evidence to suggest that permanent changes in eating habit can be brought about by the use of drugs, formula diets, or starvation. Weight loss, however, is only one aspect in the overall management of the obese, many of whom may benefit from sympathetic support and thereby learn to live with their obesity just as a dyspeptic may learn to live with his ulcer.

REFERENCES

1 Somar, E, and Sneh, E, *American Journal of Clinical Nutrition*, 1973, **25**, 845.
2 Garrow, J S, *Proceedings of the International Congress on Obesity*, p 301. London, Newman, 1975.
3 Stunkard, A J, *Archives of General Psychiatry*, 1972, **26**, 361.
4 Munro, J F, *British Journal of Hospital Medicine*, 1973, **10**, (1), 8.
5 Silverstone, J T, *Obesity; Its Pathogenesis and Management*, ch 6. Lancaster, Medical Technical Press, 1975.
6 Steel, J M, and Briggs, M, *British Medical Journal*, 1972, **3**, 26.
7 Schwartz, L N, *Journal of International Medical Research*, 1975, **3**, 328.
8 Smith, R G, Innes, J A, and Munro, J F, *British Medical Journal*, 1975, **3**, 284.
9 Chandler, J G, *Postgraduate Medicine*, 1974, **56**, 124.
10 Brewer, C, White, H, and Baddeley, M, *British Medical Journal*, 1974, **4**, 314.

Treatment of infertility and menopausal symptoms

ARNOLD KLOPPER

TREATMENT OF INFERTILITY ASSOCIATED WITH ANOVULATION

The development of effective treatment has a marvellously encouraging effect on the incidence of a disease. When, as has happened with the occasional spectacular overkill of gonadotrophin treatment of infertility, the media takes an intense interest in the treatment, the number of patients seeking it rises still more steeply. There are, however, more worthy reasons for the rising pressure. The large number of abortions has greatly reduced the availability of babies for adoption and forced would-be parents to exhaust every possibility of having a child of their own. Oral contraceptives have contributed a new cause of infertility by way of post-pill amenorrhoea, and failure of ovulation may now be simply and securely diagnosed by a single, judiciously timed plasma progesterone assay.

Good infertility clinics practise a strict investigative routine, and the existence of simple, effective treatment for one form of infertility is no good reason for short-circuiting such a routine. At the least it must be established by seminal analysis that the husband is fertile and by tubal insufflation that the wife has patent Fallopian tubes. In addition, anovulation needs to be proved. In the case of women with secondary amenorrhoea this may be taken for granted but primary amenorrhoea warrants much more extensive investigation of its own accord. Even with secondary amenorrhoea overt disease should be excluded. Occasionally the cause of anovulation is untreatable—such as menopause praecox. This condition is a likely cause of infertility when amenorrhoea is accompanied by high levels of follicle-stimulating hormone (FSH) in the blood or urine. Few doctors have not fallen into the trap of an unsuspected pregnancy. Investigation of the infertile couple needs in the first instance to go no further than establishing that the husband is fertile and that the wife has patent tubes and is not menopausal, hyperprolactinaemic, or pregnant. Because of the implications for treatment oligomenorrhoeic women should have plasma FSH and plasma prolactin assays done whenever these are available. If these investigations prove negative amenorrhoea or oligomenorrhoea is sufficient evidence of anovulation or infrequent ovulation to warrant an attempt to induce ovulation with antioestrogens.

Antioestrogens

The most commonly used antioestrogen is clomiphene citrate,

although others (notably tamoxifen in Britain) are coming into use. These compounds lead to the increased secretion of pituitary gonadotrophin by stimulating the release of the hypothalamic gonadotrophin-releasing factor. As ovulation is produced by the same endogenous endocrine events as in the normal cycle, the use of antioestrogens seldom results in overstimulation or multiple pregnancy. Indeed, there is no strong reason why their use should be confined to specialist infertility clinics. Although tamoxifen is used in smaller doses than clomiphene, the toxicity of both is so low that this is of no consequence. The standard regimen is to give clomiphene citrate 50 mg twice a day or tamoxifen 10 mg twice a day by mouth for four days. In successful cases this starts the growth of a Graafian follicle, which releases an ovum about 10 days after the start of treatment. Intercourse should therefore take place around this time. If ovulation but not conception occurs the patient will have a menstrual period three to four weeks after the start of treatment.

It is necessary to try to ascertain whether ovulation has taken place. The simplest way is by recording the basal temperature before getting up in the morning. The progesterone produced by the corpus luteum causes a sustained rise in the second half of the cycle, often as much as 0·2–0·3°C. Now that the assay of plasma progesterone is widely available assay of a single blood specimen three weeks after starting the antioestrogen will tell with certainty whether ovulation has taken place. Because chorionic gonadotrophin will cause a mature follicle to ovulate and will stimulate progesterone production by the corpus luteum the treatment with an antioestrogen is sometimes combined with an intramuscular injection of 5000 IU of chorionic gonadotrophin 10 days after starting the tablets. There is little evidence that such adjuvant treatment substantially improves the chance of a pregnancy.

If the first two or three courses of clomiphene or tamoxifen do not induce ovulation it is worth doubling the dose. If this also fails gonadotrophin treatment might be contemplated. This is quite a different kettle of fish and should not be embarked on lightly. A second round of investigation—FSH assay, prolactin assay, dynamic tests of ovarian function, and laparoscopy—should be considered. It is not appropriate here to consider in any depth the investigation and treatment of secondary amenorrhoea, which really arises at this stage. For the treatment of infertility it must be established that the woman has ovaries capable of responding to direct stimulation and a genital tract sufficiently developed to permit the meeting of the gametes and the full growth of the conceptus. This treatment is too dangerous and requires too many resources for it to be undertaken on an empirical basis.

Pituitary gonadotrophins

Human gonadotrophins are species-specific proteins and no adequate synthetic or animal substitutes are available. The FSH component may be extracted directly from human pituitaries or from menopausal urine, where it is present in relatively high concentration. Some countries, notably Australia, have organised national programmes for preparing FSH from necropsy material, and one or two large clinics in Britain also work up human pituitaries for their own use, but the only preparations commercially available are the urinary extracts Pergonal and Humegon. Although these are used primarily to induce follicular growth, the extracts contain a good deal of luteinising hormone as well as FSH, and the ovarian response is monitored by measuring the rising output of oestrogen in blood or urine. The dose needed to evoke the desired response is critical and varies from patient to patient, so that monitoring by hormone assay is mandatory, both to avoid overstimulation and to determine when a follicle mature enough to ovulate is present.

In the normal menstrual cycle ovulation is precipitated by a surge of luteinising hormone. Fortunately human chorionic gonadotrophin has a similar action and is widely available. A single injection of 5000 IU of chorionic gonadotrophin will cause the follicle, stimulated to the right stage of development by the FSH injections, to ovulate some 36 hours after the human chorionic gonadotrophin injection. Unfortunately even a slight overdose of FSH will cause numerous follicles to develop and all will be ovulated by the human chorionic gonadotrophin. The litters that may result from such an unhappy therapeutic accident have been one of medicine's less fortunate contributions to the lay press.

Ergot alkaloids

A third therapeutic agent has lately joined antioestrogens and pituitary gonadotrophins. In some anovulatory, generally amenorrhoeic women the menstrual irregularity is accompanied by excess prolactin production from the anterior pituitary. Such hyperprolactinaemia may be suppressed by various ergot alkaloids, notably bromocriptine. Even in the absence of demonstrable prolactin excess this compound may induce ovulation. At present it is still basking in a rising sun, but, although its eventual role may be smaller than is presently assigned to it by enthusiasts, it is undoubtedly an important addition to the therapeutic armamentarium against failure of ovulation.

Luteinising hormone-releasing hormone

Many ovulation-inducing agents act by liberating luteinising hormone-releasing hormone (LH-RH) from the hypothalamus. The constitution of this decapeptide is now known. It has been synthesised and is commercially available. At first glance this appears to be the logical way to treat anovulation so long as the pituitary is intact and able to respond. As an agent for inducing ovulation LH-RH has proved disappointing for physiological reasons that were obvious from the start. LH-RH has a short half life in the circulation and is destroyed within a few minutes. Under normal physiological conditions it has only a few centimetres to travel from the hypothalamus to the target organ, the pituitary. It does so dissolved in a few millilitres of blood. Once past the pituitary it is greatly diluted and rapidly removed. Treatment necessarily starts by administering the polypeptide into the general circulation, and very little reaches the pituitary. To achieve sufficient gonadotrophin release to cause ovulation LH-RH has to be administered often and in high doses over a long time. Although the use of the natural material is thus impracticable, many experiments with analogues, less easily metabolised, are under way, and it may be that one of these will give us mastery over releasing gonadotrophins from the pituitary.

Ethinyloestradiol

Other attempts to imitate the physiological signals causing gonadotrophin release have met with modest and unpredictable success. The growing Graafian follicle secretes increasing amounts of oestradiol. The rising oestrogen concentration is the physiological feedback control of the hypothalamus. When the oestrogen reaches a critical level LH-RH is liberated and causes a surge of luteinising hormone, which immediately precedes ovulation. It is sometimes possible in an amenorrhoeic woman producing little oestrogen to imitate this positive oestrogen feedback by giving small doses of ethinyloestradiol or oestradiol-17β. This treatment, although it has the attraction of simplicity and safety, is so much less predictable than other means of inducing ovulation that it is seldom used.

HORMONAL TREATMENT OF MENOPAUSAL SYMPTOMS

Although effective endocrine agents for suppressing the unpleasant manifestations of the climacteric have been known for nearly 50 years, they have been used on a large scale only in the past decade. Even today their widespread use is more a matter of social pressure than medical enterprise. As is often the case, the wave of therapeutic enthusiasm started in the United States. Some of the more extravagant claims—"no woman need have a menopause"—may be discounted, but it is proper that we should respond to the needs of our patients even when these are voiced in the lay press with more force than wisdom. The question is not whether general practitioners should prescribe endocrine preparations and hospitals create hormone-replacement clinics. We are already too far down that path to turn back. The problem is how to control the traffic: how to select patients, what preparations to give, and when to stop.

Hot flushes

The menopause presents a whole constellation of symptoms—loss of libido, insomnia, headaches, hot flushes, atrophic vaginitis, and a lot more besides. It is therapeutic nonsense to attack them all with a barrage of medicines. By and large the commonest and most troublesome manifestation is hot flushes, and treatment should be directed at it. Fortunately the effect of treatment may be evaluated objectively by a flush count. Because of insomnia, restlessness, and depression, hypnotics or sedatives are sometimes combined with hormones in proprietary preparations. This approach should be eschewed. In the few cases when such symptoms altogether outweigh the flushes they should be treated in their own right. Androgens such as testosterone are protein anabolics. They may give a feeling of wellbeing, increase appetite, increase weight, and improve libido. They are not a specific treatment for the ill effects of the menopause. Menopausal women are naturally prone to hirsuties. When the growth of a moustache coincides with taking androgens the doctor may be unjustly blamed. On the whole, androgens are best avoided.

Oestrogen replacement

The principal endocrine change of the menopause is that the ovaries cease to secrete oestradiol. The postmenopausal woman is not altogether deprived of oestrogen. Some oestrone is made by the peripheral conversion of androstenedione but not enough to prevent the consequences of oestrogen deprivation—namely, bone and skin changes and vascular instability. Treatment in the menopause should replace the missing oestrogen. To this end many compounds are available, mostly synthetic, and different from the 22 oestrogens that have been isolated from the biological fluids of pregnant women. A third category are oestrogens such as equilin and equilenin, which, although isolated from other mammals, do not occur in man. The most commonly used artificial oestrogens are ethinyloestradiol, mestranol, and stilboestrol. The liver and other tissues have an array of enzymes that metabolise and inactivate oestrogens in various ways, so that any natural oestrogen not taken up by target organs is rapidly disposed of. The synthetic oestrogens are metabolised much more slowly and owe their potency and perhaps their toxicity to the physiological mechanisms for their inactivation being much less efficient.

Many untoward effects have been ascribed to synthetic oestrogens. Their tendency to cause thrombosis and to affect carbohydrate tolerance deleteriously has been well documented. The problem of whether synthetic oestrogens can cause cancer is unresolved. In a few particular instances the evidence is strong—for instance, cancer of the vagina in girls resulting from the antenatal treatment of their mothers with artificial oestrogens. In the context of menopausal treatment much disquiet has been aroused by the apparent association between endometrial carcinoma and the use of so-called "natural" oestrogens from equine sources.

The evidence against the natural oestrogens—oestrone, oestradiol, and oestriol—is less strong. Therapeutically they have the disadvantage that when taken by mouth they are rapidly inactivated before they reach the target organs. This has been overcome by preparing combinations, generally fatty-acid esters, that hydrolyse slowly in the body, yielding the free oestrogen. Oestrone and oestradiol benzoate are old familiars. To these, more advanced preparations (such as oestradiol valerate and oestrone piperazine sulphate) have lately been added. Oestriol, an impeded oestrogen, is worth special consideration. It binds to the oestrogen receptor in the cytoplasm of the cells of oestrogen-responsive tissues and is conveyed to the nucleus, where it sets in train the cascade of events leading to fresh protein synthesis and cell replication. It is, however, less strongly bound than oestradiol and tends to escape from the cell before the whole sequence is completed. Although it will cause vaginal cornification and suppress hot flushes (both desirable effects in menopausal women), it is not a strong stimulus to endometrial proliferation and seldom causes postmenopausal bleeding. In so far as menopausal treatment is aimed at replacing lost ovarian secretion, it is logical to use oestradiol—the very material produced by the ovary. In summary, oestriol 0·5–1·0 mg daily or oestradiol valerate or oestrone sulphate up to 2 mg daily is the first choice.

Whether to give hormone replacement treatment to menopausal women and when to stop are matters of nice judgment. To some degree, as earlier with pain-killers in labour, our attitudes are socially not medically conditioned. In face of the strength of public demand our apparent choice is to some extent deceptive. A reasonable course between Scylla and Charybdis is to treat those who ask for it but not to push it and to use such agents as will relieve our patients without exposing them to undue risk.

Diseases of the cardiovascular system

Drugs affecting the cardiovascular system: pharmacological basis of treatment

JOHN C GILBERT

The functioning of the heart and blood vessels can be influenced by many drugs, and a wide variety of mechanisms is implicated in the drugs' actions. This account will be heavily restricted, but will cover many drugs used clinically.

CARDIAC GLYCOSIDES

The cardiac glycosides slow the heart in atrial fibrillation and also increase the force of contraction of the heart by increasing the rate at which tension is developed. This increases the cardiac output and increases blood flow to other organs, including the kidneys—where water excretion is enhanced. Observations in animals and man indicate that digitalis acts directly on contractility. If the heart is of normal size the net cardiac output need not be increased. If the heart is failing, however, its efficiency is depressed and by its positive inotropic effect digitalis restores this and increases the output.

The increased contractility and cardiac output induce a response in baroreceptor activity, and this results in increased vagal activity and slowing of the heart. This contributes to the beneficial effect of digitalis in atrial fibrillation. Other events are also implicated, however, particularly a direct action on the atrioventricular node so that the effective or functional refractory period is prolonged; this reduces the frequency of ventricular contraction. But these effects of digitalis may also underlie some of its toxic manifestations, which include estrasystoles, usually arising in the ventricles; atrial and ventricular tachycardias; and heart block.

Speculation concerning the mechanism of the positive inotropic action of digitalis has centred mainly on the role of adenosine triphosphatase (ATPase), which is activated by sodium and potassium ions together (Na,K-ATPase) in the presence of magnesium ions. This enzyme is present in the membrane of the heart cell, and its function is to mediate the pumping of sodium ions out of the cell and potassium ions into the cell against concentration gradients, the energy for these processes being supplied by the splitting of adenosine triphosphate. Some 20 years ago it was shown that this enzyme is strongly inhibited by cardiac glycosides. Such inhibition interferes with the coupled sodium-potassium pump, and sodium ions accumulate in the heart muscle cell.

Much evidence suggests that glycosides that do not inhibit the enzyme do not exert a positive inotropic effect on the heart: digitalis does not exert this effect in species where it fails to inhibit ATPase.

These observations support the hypothesis that the effect of digitalis on heart contractility is mediated through inhibition of the ATPase. Some studies, however, have thrown doubt on this relationship and on the fundamental concept that this enzyme is the receptor for the drug in the heart. For instance, while some experiments have shown a direct relation between wash-out of the pharmacological action of digitalis in the isolated animal heart and the dissociation of the drug from Na,K-ATPase preparations, others have suggested that inhibition of the enzyme may persist after the decay of the positive inotropic effect. The problem is complicated by the role of ions, such as calcium, other than sodium and potassium in the heart cell. When the muscle cell membrane depolarises, calcium ions enter the cell. Moreover, calcium is released from bound forms within the cell so that the contractile mechanism is activated. In relaxation the released calcium is taken up again by membrane systems and also calcium moves out of the cell. There is evidence that links the inward movement of calcium, which initiates the contractile process, with the inward movement of sodium ions.

Putting these ideas together one can postulate that cardiac glycosides inhibit the Na,K-ATPase, causing sodium to enter the cell. This triggers the entry of calcium ions (which may, however, be independent of sodium ion entry) and increases the availability of this ion to the contractile machinery. Despite evidence to the contrary, therefore—and despite a hypothesis suggesting that digitalis in low concentrations mediates its effects on the heart by actually stimulating the ATPase—the positive inotropic action so vital for alleviating congestive heart failure may result from ATPase inhibition.

Whatever the mechanism of the therapeutic action of digitalis, one is on firmer ground in proposing that the toxic manifestations of drug treatment result from inhibition of ATPase. Digitalis and potassium ions compete for a site on the outside of the membrane where potassium normally increases enzymic activity, and this results in enzyme inhibition. Because the process includes competition the effect of the drug may be increased by decreasing the serum potassium concentration. Hence diuretics that cause hypokalaemia have to be used carefully. Nevertheless, recent work suggests that some potassium-sparing diuretics may raise the threshold of digoxin toxicity by a direct action on the heart rather than on the kidney. This action could result if the drugs directly inhibit the loss of potassium from the heart muscle cell.

Diuretics play a prominent part in treating heart failure not accompanied by fibrillation, and they are also added to the therapeutic regimen after digoxin treatment when fibrillation does occur.

ANTIARRHYTHMIC DRUGS

Quinidine was introduced as an antiarrhythmic agent after the observation that atrial fibrillation in patients with malaria who were treated with quinine or quinidine was considerably improved. Since then the antiarrhythmic action has been investigated using electrophysiological techniques and several factors are now known to be involved in its action and in the actions of other antiarrhythmics. Four basic mechanisms have been proposed, and several of these may be responsible for the final action of any one drug: (*a*) stabilisation of the membrane, (*b*) interference with the influence on the heart of the sympathetic nervous system, (*c*) increase in the duration of the cardiac action potential, and (*d*) interference with inward calcium currents.

Quinidine raises the threshold potential—the potential at which the degree of depolarisation of the membrane triggers an action potential. It also increases the effective refractory period (a period in the cardiac cycle when an impulse cannot be propagated) both by reducing the rate of depolarisation (reducing the action potential duration) and by prolonging the repolarisation process. This decreases the heart rate, and it appears to be the basis for the past use of both quinidine and procainamide in atrial fibrillation.

Phenytoin, in contrast to quinidine, decreases the effective refractory period. It is not used in atrial fibrillation but it does counteract digitalis-induced tachycardia. The drug increases the rate of rise of the action potential and decreases the action potential duration (again in contrast to quinidine). Membrane responsiveness is increased and conduction improved. This is believed to reduce the chance of conduction block and of spasmodic or recurrent re-entrant rhythms—rhythms occurring when an impulse that has been blocked along one path through the tissue is permitted to re-enter by another and so to precipitate a premature contraction or arrythmia.

Lignocaine is another commonly used antiarrhythmic, particularly for ventricular arrhythmias. It reduces the duration of the action potential and as a result the effective refractory period: action potential ratio is increased in the Purkinje fibres and the muscle fibres so that the discharge at "ectopic foci" is opposed. This means that spontaneous depolarisation at foci some distance from those sites normally responsible for pacemaker activity is prevented from intruding on such activity. Beta-adrenergic receptor antagonists such as practolol and propranolol have also been useful in treating arrhythmias. Whether the value of propranolol depends more on its quinidine-like action which results in membrane stabilisation or on its beta-adrenoceptor antagonist activity is difficult to say. While the beta-receptor antagonist activity is pronounced in the (−)- but not the (+)-isomer of propranolol, antiarrhythmic activity is pronounced in both, suggesting that membrane stabilisation is important. Even so, low doses of (−)-propranolol are said to be effective in treating paroxysmal tachycardias, and we know that noradrenaline can induce depolarisation at ectopic foci and cause an arrhythmia.

VASODILATORS

Since amylnitrite was introduced in 1867 for treating angina several nitrites have been examined for pharmacological activity and they remain the most important vasodilators for this condition. They are effective because they cause quite non-specific relaxation of smooth muscle. The heat relies on a continuous supply of oxygen from the blood, and any impairment of the efficiency of the coronary circulation must be corrected quickly.

Glyceryl trinitrate increases the coronary blood flow in normal vessels, but whether this is because of dilatation of the coronary vessels is not known. The response of diseased vessels is quite another matter. Possibly the larger coronary vessels become dilated but there is considerable doubt as to the response of smaller vessels. Moreover, possibly any decrease in coronary resistance is too short to account for the alleviation of angina. Probably the decreased venous return caused by nitrites and the resulting reduced diastolic volume of the ventricles are important actions because the work performed by the heart is reduced. Drugs such as theophylline and its ethylenediamine derivative aminophylline have pronounced coronary vasodilator action in normal vessels but they are toxic and so have not been used routinely in treating angina.

ANTIHYPERTENSIVE DRUGS

The most commonly used drugs in treating hypertension are diuretics, particularly the thiazides. The direct effects of the drugs on vascular smooth muscle may well be concerned in their action.

Vascular smooth-muscle relaxants

Drugs that relax vascular smooth muscle are gaining importance in treating hypertension because they decrease the resistance of the peripheral vascular bed. We still do not know how this relaxant activity occurs, though hydrallazine, for example, appears to affect arterioles more than veins. Diazoxide is a potent antihypertensive drug that, though structurally similar to the thiazide diuretics, is not a diuretic. Diazoxide is particularly useful in the emergency treatment of hypertension: given intravenously, it has a direct effect on vascular smooth muscle that results in vasodilatation and a rapid fall in blood pressure. Again, it affects the arterioles more than the veins but we do not know the precise mechanism. If it antagonises the effects of calcium ions, as has been suggested, then its powerful vasodilator action could result from interference with the role of calcium in generating action potentials or in the release of calcium ions during the initiation of muscle contraction.

Several antihypertensive agents affect sympathetic nerves and adrenergic receptors. The constrictor action of noradrenaline, released from sympathetic nerves, on vascular smooth muscle can be antagonised by alpha-adrenergic antagonists such as phentolamine.

Pentolinium has an antihypertensive action by blocking transmission in sympathetic ganglia, but the drug is now seldom used. Adrenergic neurone-blocking drugs such as guanethidine, bethanidine, and debrisoquine are also used as antihypertensive agents. These act in a third way: after they are taken up into the adrenergic nerve terminal they prevent the release of noradrenaline.

Beta-adrenergic antagonists

Beta-adrenergic antagonists such as propranolol are of value for treating hypertension, and they may be given with vasodilators. The onset of the antihypertensive effect of propranolol is not immediate, and the mechanism of its action is still not clear, though its role in reducing the heart rate and the cardiac output is obviously important. Propranolol also affects the peripheral blood vessels and lowers the plasma renin activity. The latter action would lower angiotensin levels, and since angiotensin contracts vascular smooth muscle, the result would be a reduction of the peripheral vascular resistance.

Two other possible mechanisms of propranolol are a change in the sensitivity of the baroreceptors of the carotid sinus and major arteries, so that their performance adjusts to the reduced cardiac output, and a direct effect on the central nervous system.

Methyldopa

Methyldopa has been one of the main antihypertensive agents for some years, but recently the mechanism for this action has been re-examined and an effect on the central nervous system (CNS) now appears to be implicated. There is little doubt that methyldopa is an inhibitor of dopadecarboxylase, the enzyme converting dopa (dihydroxyphenylalanine) to dopamine. This depresses the synthesis both of dopamine itself and of noradrenaline and in addition, since 5-hydroxytryptamine decarboxylase is also susceptible to inhibition by methyldopa, serotonin (5-hydroxytryptamine) synthesis is also decreased. The depression of noradrenaline synthesis, in particular, seemed to provide a good basis for the antihypertensive action of methyldopa in view of the effect of the catecholamine of increasing the resistance of the peripheral vascular bed through a vasoconstrictor action mediated via alpha-adrenoceptors. Depletion of noradrenaline, however, does not appear to follow the same time-course as the antihypertensive action of methyldopa and in addition alpha-methyldopamine, which also inhibits dopadecarboxylase, has little antihypertensive effect. It has recently been observed that dopadecarboxylase inhibitors that penetrate the CNS nullify the antihypertensive effect of methyldopa, whereas inhibitors of the enzyme acting outside the CNS do not. A hypothesis compatible with these observations is that methyldopa acts not at the periphery but in the CNS where it is metabolised to alpha-methylnoradrenaline; this compound may exert an antihypertensive action through interaction with central alpha-adrenoceptors.

Clonidine

A drug often used in mild hypertension is clonidine, though initially it may increase the blood pressure. This may reflect the fact that clonidine, which is structurally similar to tolazoline, the alpha-adrenoceptor antagonist, has intrinsic alpha-adrenoceptor agonist activity so that a direct but transient peripheral vasoconstrictor action could occur. Its withdrawal may cause rebound hypertension.

The adrenoceptor agonist activity may be concerned also in its antihypertensive action if alpha-adrenoceptors in the CNS are activated so that the sympathetic nervous system is inhibited. This hypothesis is a difficult one to test but the action of clonidine does seem to result from effects in the CNS rather than at the periphery.

One cannot include here a discussion of the mechanisms of all the drugs that influence the activity of the cardiovascular system. Those which have been mentioned, however, do illustrate the extent to which the treatment of cardiovascular disorders has a sound pharmacological basis.

Hypertension

J C PETRIE

The Framingham study has shown that the risk of cardiovascular "events" rises in proportion to the height of the blood pressure, systolic or diastolic, with no discernible critical level.[1] Such evidence has been taken to suggest that an active reduction of blood pressure is desirable. The Framingham study and much life insurance information, however, is concerned with the natural history of a population with a wide range of blood pressures. These studies offer minimal information about the effects of antihypertensive treatment.

The outstanding evidence for the beneficial effects of drug treatment comes from carefully controlled Veterans Administration studies.[2-5] In men with sustained diastolic blood pressure readings above 110 mm Hg (phase 4*) antihypertensive treatment resulted in a reduction of severe morbid events associated with hypertension, such as congestive cardiac failure, renal failure, and stroke. Unfortunately no reduction in the complications of coronary artery disease was shown. In women other than with severe hypertension the influence of hypotensive treatment has not been clearly established. At diastolic blood pressures below 110 mm Hg (phase 4) the case for treatment is not proved, and large-scale multicentre trials are in progress to determine the effects of reduction of blood pressure in patients with mild hypertension and in the elderly. In such patients the decision to start treatment should not be based on a solitary high reading, systolic or diastolic. The blood pressure should be measured on at least three separate occasions at weekly or two-weekly intervals, as a significant fall in blood pressure readings occurs without drug treatment over this period if the measurement is made under similar circumstances by the same observer. Ideally a profile of casual, lying or sitting (3–5 min), standing (1–3 min), and post-exercise blood pressure levels should be obtained on each occasion, preferably at different times of day. The diastolic end-point should be recorded as phase 4 or phase 5 or both. Care to eliminate factors that may distort the measurement must also be taken.[6] For example, the width and length of cuff for the sphygmomanometer varies in relation to the size of the arm (childhood or obesity), and the rate of deflation of the cuff should be steady and slow (2–3 mm/s fall in the column of mercury).

The decision to start treatment—for example, in a 40-year-old man with a sustained lying blood pressure of 165/100 mm Hg (phase 4)—is also weighted by proved "risk" factors, such as raised lipid values,

* Phase 4, distinct, abrupt muffling of sound; phase 5, disappearance of sounds.

cigarette smoking, glucose intolerance, and electrocardiographic evidence of left ventricular hypertrophy.[1] A strong family history of cardiovascular events or features thought to be associated with sustained high blood pressure such as cardiac hypertrophy, renal damage, or fundal changes are further indications that treatment should be started, even though the benefits of antihypertensive treatment at this level of blood pressure in a 40-year-old man have to be proved. In women, who appear to tolerate raised blood pressure levels better than men, or in obese or older patients, the arguments for active treatment at a level of 165/100mm Hg are much weaker. Only enthusiastic believers in the benefits of active reduction of minor increases in blood pressure would initiate treatment.

The decision to treat is also influenced by the presence of underlying causes of hypertension. Examples include concurrent drug treatment such as oral contraceptives or corticosteroids, primary aldosteronism, coarctation of the aorta, Cushing's syndrome, and phaeochromocytoma. Age, occupation, and personality of the patient also affect the decision.

Clearly a rigid policy not to treat any patient with casual, lying, or standing baseline levels below 110 mm Hg is untenable. Similarly critical examination must be made of exhortations to start treatment in all patients with a diastolic level above 90 mm Hg. Indeed, such a casual diastolic blood pressure may be found in 20–30% of adults.

WHAT TO USE

Mild and moderate levels of hypertension are usually symptomless at diagnosis. Patients will persevere with lifelong treatment only if it does not interfere too much with their daily activities. In clinical practice most grades of hypertension may be treated satisfactorily with a limited number of drugs—at most six—chosen from the 90 preparations marketed in Britain. These can be used alone or in various combinations.

DIURETICS

Diuretics (23 preparations) and diuretic combinations (25 preparations) are widely used for all grades of hypertension. There is no evidence of a clear superiority of any individual benzothiadiazine diuretic. The mode of action of thiazides in long-term treatment is uncertain. An effect on vascular smooth muscle, perhaps mediated through a reduction in intracellular sodium and water, has been suggested. The onset of hypotensive action is within two to three days but may not be fully developed even after four weeks of treatment. The once-daily dose required (say bendrofluazide 5 mg/day) is below that needed to produce a troublesome diuresis, and the use of high-potency diuretics such as frusemide or bumetanide offers no advantage. Longer-acting diuretics such as chlorthalidone or aldosterone antagonists such as spironolactone are also effective. The mean reduction in sustained lying and standing blood pressures obtained with bendrofluazide 5 mg/day under controlled conditions is 15–20 mm Hg systolic and 5–10 mm Hg diastolic. Combined treatment with other agents such as beta-blockers or methyldopa is rational as an increased hypotensive effect is obtained.

The principal adverse reactions to thiazide diuretics include rashes, mild gastrointestinal symptoms, hypokalaemia, impairment of glucose tolerance, raised serum urate levels, and aggravation of renal insufficiency. Potassium supplements are seldom required in patients on a normal daily diet containing over 70 mmol (mEq) potassium if low doses of thiazide diuretics are used—such as bendrofluazide 5 mg/day. In potassium-losing states or when there is doubt about the dietary intake and in patients with impaired liver function or receiving concurrent treatment with digoxin, corticosteroids, or carbenoxolone, potassium supplements (24–32 mmol/day) or a potassium-sparing or retaining diuretic are indicated. Diabetes mellitus is not an absolute contraindication to thiazides. Alterations in antidiabetic treatment, diet, and exercise may counteract any adverse effect of the diuretic on glucose tolerance. Newer agents, such as metolazone, are reputed to cause less deterioration in glucose handling. Allopurinol may be prescribed in patients who develop hyperuricaemia secondary to thiazide treatment, although other antihypertensive agents such as beta-blockers may be preferred. Photosensitivity and thrombocytopenia are among other adverse effects that have been reported. Raised plasma renin levels have been associated with an adverse prognosis in hypertension, although the evidence is controversial. Thiazides raise renin levels, and their use in hypertension has been questioned on theoretical grounds.

BETA-ADRENOCEPTOR ANTAGONISTS

Eight proprietary beta-blockers (six drugs) are marketed in Britain. The use of beta-blockers as first-choice treatment either alone or in combination with other agents is increasing. Possession of partial agonist (intrinsic sympathomimetic), cardioselective, or local anaesthetic (quinidine-like or membrane-stabilising) activity has not been shown to confer antihypertensive superiority.

Differences occur in the handling of different beta-blockers—for example, absorption (propranolol, almost complete; oxprenolol 70–100%); protein binding (propranolol 90–95%; metoprolol 12%); volume of distribution (practolol 1·6, propranolol 3·6, metoprolol 5·6 l/kg); formation of active metabolic products and urinary excretion of unchanged drug (oxprenolol 22–29%; propranolol 1–4%). In addition, wide inter-individual variations in response complicate the interpretation of the effects of single and repeated fixed doses of beta-blockers such as propranolol. Throughout the dosage range the mode of action in reducing blood pressure remains controversial. Speculation continues about the relative contributions of the fall in cardiac output (variable), fall in peripheral resistance (variable), and central and baroreceptor influences as well as the effects of the renin-angiotensin axis (variable reduction in renin release).

The optimal starting and maintenance doses and the time of onset of hypotensive action of beta-blockers are not clearly established. Higher and less frequent initial oral doses—for example, 40 or 80 mg propranolol or oxprenolol two or three times a day—are now being recommended than when beta-blockers were introduced over 10 years ago. A reduction of pressure within four hours with such doses is usually obtained. No further reductions in blood pressure occur after two weeks on a fixed dose, and a two-fold increase in dose is usually recommended. A twice-daily dosage regimen appears to be satisfactory with some agents—for example, propranolol and oxprenolol. About a fifth of the patients do not respond to conventional doses of beta-blockers (say, propranolol 240–320 mg/day). In such non-responders alternative hypotensive treatment may be added or substituted, although some workers have increased the dose of beta-blockers to 2–5 g/day, at which levels a central mode of action may assume an increased importance. The mean reduction in supine and erect blood pressure under controlled conditions in a randomly selected group of patients is about 20/10 mm Hg with propranolol 120–240 mg/day. Once such a reduction has been obtained, doubling the dose of beta-blocker—for example, atenolol (above 100 mg/day) or oxprenolol (above 360–480 mg/day)—may not cause further significant reduction. Combination treatment with other drugs such as thiazides is effective.

The predictable pharmacological actions of beta-blockers imply that their use is contraindicated in patients with asthma, moderate and severe heart failure, conduction defects (2° and 3°), metabolic acidosis, and prolonged fasting. Relative contraindications quoted by some manufacturers include chronic obstructive lung disease, severe cardiomegaly, mild cardiac failure, pregnancy, allergic rhinitis, diabetes mellitus, and sinus bradycardia. In these instances the potential benefits of beta-blockade must be weighed against the disadvantages.

Many adverse reactions have been associated with beta-blockers. Nausea, anorexia, and vomiting may be reduced by taking them before food. A rise in blood urea levels and deterioration in renal function have been reported as with other hypotensive agents. On the other hand, successful use of beta-blockers and a reduction in the plasma half life of propranolol have also been described in renal failure. The avoidance of high doses (say, over 400 mg propranolol or oxprenolol daily) may reduce the occurrence of symptoms of mild fatigue, lassitude, lightheadedness, ataxia, anxiety, mental confusion, hallucinations, insomnia, vivid dreams, and a hypertensive response, which have been reported in some patients. In cold climates, cold extremities, aggravation of Raynaud's phenomenon, and symptoms of peripheral vascular disease may be troublesome. Rashes have been reported with most agents. Several minor adverse reactions have also been described. In severe ischaemic heart disease withdrawal of beta-blockers should not be abrupt, as deaths from cardiac arrhythmia and myocardial infarction have been reported. The principal adverse drug interaction concerns antidiabetic treatment. Signs of hypoglycaemia may be masked and the hypoglycaemic effects of concurrent treatment increased.

A validated case of the oculomucocutaneous syndrome associated with practolol treatment has not yet been reported with any other beta-blocker. Careful monitoring of patients on beta-blockers, particularly the newer agents, is required. The cause of the reaction has not been determined. Investigations are in progress to determine possible immunological, chemical, or genetic factors.

METHYLDOPA

The use of low doses of methyldopa (500–750 mg/day) either alone or in combination with other drugs reduces the troublesome adverse effects, such as drowsiness, that occasionally limit its usefulness as a single drug used in high doses (2 g/day or more). The explanation of the mode of action has undergone considerable change. The main hypotensive action of methyldopa is now believed to be mediated through the action of a metabolite, perhaps α-methylnoradrenaline, on the central nervous system to stimulate central alpha-receptors rather than through peripheral effects. Methyldopa also lowers renin activity.

An appreciable reduction in blood pressure may be obtained within three to six hours in the bedfast patient if a high initial oral dose (750–1000 mg) is used. Such doses are rarely employed because rapid and dramatic reduction of blood pressure is indicated only in the severest grades of hypertension. Furthermore, the starting of methyldopa treatment is often delayed because it interferes with the estimation of catecholamines to show a false-positive reaction in the screening test for phaeochromocytoma. Used in conventional doses (500–3000 mg/day) methyldopa reduces supine, erect, and post-exercise blood pressures. Few carefully controlled comparative studies have been carried out but it appears that the hypotensive efficacy is at least equivalent to that of beta-blockers, adrenergic neurone blockers, and clonidine. When added to other hypotensive agents a lower starting dose (375–500 mg/day) should be used and the dose of the other agent also reduced until the effectiveness of the combination can be assessed. If a further hypotensive effect is required or tolerance develops increases in doses are usually by 250 mg increments at intervals of two to three days, preferably at night because of possible sedation. Methyldopa is largely excreted by the kidney and smaller doses are recommended in renal insufficiency. A rise in blood urea may occur during treatment as with other antihypertensive agents. There is no clear evidence that methyldopa regularly reduces the renal glomerular filtration rate in hypertensive patients. Indeed, glomerular filtration is usually maintained or even increased.

Methyldopa is contraindicated in hepatitis and active cirrhosis and is not recommended in patients with a history of liver disease. Jaundice, hepatocellular damage, cholestasis, and abnormal liver function values have been reported. In 10 to 20% of patients a positive reaction to the direct Coombs test develops, usually within 12 months of starting treatment. An association has been shown with doses greater than 1 g/day. The Coombs test result becomes negative within months of stopping methyldopa. An acquired haemolytic anaemia associated with methyldopa treatment is another uncommon reason for stopping it. Reversible effects on white blood cells, especially granulocytes, have been reported in a few cases. The most common adverse reactions are drowsiness, sedation, failure of concentration, and weakness, especially during the initial period of treatment. Some patients cannot tolerate even low doses. Gastrointestinal disturbance, drug fever, rashes, weight gain, giddiness, nightmares, depression, dryness of the mouth, nasal congestion, sexual dysfunction, non-puerperal lactation, and Parkinsonism also occur. A paradoxical pressor response has occasionally been reported, particularly after parenteral administration.

BETHANIDINE, DEBRISOQUINE, AND GUANETHIDINE

Adrenergic neurone blockers may be used in all grades of hypertension, although some doctors reserve them for moderate or severe hypertension. In such patients the adrenergic neurone blocker is added, usually in low doses, to existing antihypertensive treatment. The selection of drug is a matter of personal preference, although bethanidine and debrisoquine appear to have some advantages over guanethidine. The mode of action of adrenergic neurone blockers is complex, and effects have been shown on the storage and release of noradrenaline. The duration of action of bethanidine (2–12 hours) and debrisoquine (4–24 hours) allows more rapid adjustments of dosage to be made than with guanethidine, which is longer-acting. On the other hand, once the optimal maintenance dose is known, more frequent daily dosage may be a disadvantage with the shorter-acting drugs and the compliance of patients with treatment may be better with debrisoquine or guanethidine given once daily.

The recommended initial dose is small (say, bethanidine 5–10 mg thrice daily, debrisoquine 10–20 mg once or twice daily) and small increments in dosage should be made at short intervals (bethanidine 1–2 days, debrisoquine 2–4 days, guanethidine 5–7 days). Assessment of effect should include measurement of the standing and preferably post-exercise blood pressure levels, because postural and post-exercise hypotension may be troublesome. Reduction of supine blood pressure is variable. In patients who prove difficult to control, more satisfactory levels of blood pressure may be achieved by combination with another hypotensive drug rather than by using high doses of adrenergic neurone blocker alone, and the occurrence of unpleasant adverse reactions may be reduced. In renal insufficiency a reduction in dosage is recommended. On the rare occasions that large and rapid reductions in blood pressure are essential and other parenteral preparations such as diazoxide, hydrallazine, clonidine, or guanethidine are not available the cautious use of a higher initial oral dose of a short-acting agent (say, bethanidine 20–30 mg) is effective in the bedfast patient.

The principal adverse reactions of adrenergic neurone blockers include postural and post-exercise hypotension, which may be troublesome in the elderly or in warm climates; diarrhoea; and aggravation of peptic ulcer symptoms, particularly in patients taking guanethidine. Failure of ejaculation, weakness, nasal stuffiness, and fluid retention may also occur. If parenteral guanethidine is indicated it should be given preferably by intramuscular injection or slow intravenous infusion, as an initial hypertensive response may occur.

The awareness of doctors of clinically important adverse drug reactions involving adrenergic neurone blockers is low. Pressor responses or a reduction of the hypotensive action may develop if concurrent treatment is prescribed. Examples include tricyclic antidepressants, sympathomimetic agents present in cold and cough cures and decongestants, monoamine oxidase inhibitors, chlorpromazine, and appetite suppressants.

CLONIDINE

Clonidine is an effective antihypertensive agent and is a useful alternative. Its mode of action is not fully understood. An alpha-adrenoceptor agonist effect has been shown, and the central hypotensive effects can be antagonised by alpha-adrenoceptor-blocking drugs such as phentolamine. In addition, a reduction in the activity of sympathetic nerves, peripheral effects on smooth muscle, and inhibition of neuronal uptake mechanisms have been shown. Clonidine reduces renin activity.

The starting dose should be low (0·15–0·3 mg/day). The maximum effect occurs two to four hours after a single dose. A thrice-daily dosage scheme is recommended, although recent pharmacokinetic studies suggest that a twice-daily regimen may be feasible. The need to take clonidine tablets regularly must be emphasised. The drug should not be discontinued abruptly—for example, around the time of emergency surgery—because sudden withdrawal of long-term oral clonidine treatment may be associated with severe "rebound" hypertensive response and symptoms of headache, anxiety, and hyperirritability. This hypertensive effect may be increased if the patient is taking beta-blockers. Pretreatment with desipramine may antagonise the hypotensive action of clonidine. After oral treatment bradycardia, sedation, reduced salivary flow, fluid retention, mild aggravation of renal insufficiency, depression, and gastrointestinal symptoms may also occur. In emergencies intravenous clonidine may be given by slow injection to minimise a transient initial rise in blood pressure that occurs in some patients.

HYDRALLAZINE

The combination of oral hydrallazine and other vasodilators such as prazosin or minoxidil with beta-blockers is useful, effective, and increasingly popular. Other agents such as thiazides or methyldopa may be added to the "cocktail" of treatment, particularly in patients with unsatisfactory levels of blood pressure. Hydrallazine has a direct effect on arteriolar smooth muscle. Used alone it reduces blood pressure, diastolic levels often more than systolic, and peripheral vascular resistance. This is associated with an increase in heart rate, stroke volume, and cardiac output and with symptoms such as palpitations, aggravation of angina, and headache, which limit its usefulness. Plasma renin activity rises. The addition of a beta-blocker, however, reduces or abolishes the apparently reflex effects such as tachycardia and increases the efficacy and acceptability to the patient of vasodilators. In addition, the combination allows lower doses of hydrallazine to be used (75–100 mg/day in three or four divided doses). Hydrallazine may also be given parenterally in hypertensive emergencies. Twenty to 40 mg should be given by slow intravenous injection.

Hydrallazine should be used with care in patients with severe ischaemic heart disease, particularly if concurrent beta-blockers are not prescribed. In some patients long-term administration of high doses—for example, 400 mg/day or more—results in an acute rheumatoid state or in a syndrome similar to systemic lupus erythematosus and treatment should be stopped. Adverse reactions may also be troublesome at low doses. These include gastrointestinal upsets, sweating, fluid retention, conjunctivitis, and nasal congestion. The metabolism of hydrallazine is partly through N-acetylation, which is under genetic control. In patients who are "slow" acetylators and in severe renal insufficiency, accumulation may develop with an associated increase in adverse effects.

DIAZOXIDE

Intravenous diazoxide should be reserved for the emergency reduction of blood pressure in hypertensive crises. The patient should be lying flat and 150–300 mg (or 5 mg/kg) should be given intravenously over 10 seconds. This usually reduces severely raised levels of blood pressure within five to 10 minutes, although further doses may be required (up to 1200 mg in 24 hours). Diazoxide is related chemically to the thiazide group. It has a direct effect on vascular smooth muscle. The amount of fall in blood pressure is unpredictable and may be hazardous in the elderly or in patients with cerebrovascular disease. Diazoxide treatment is also associated with a reflex tachycardia and fluid retention, which may be troublesome in patients with myocardial insufficiency. Concurrent diuretic treatment may be required. Diazoxide is also available as an oral hypotensive agent and has been used in patients with severe renal failure. The efficacy of oral treatment is not clearly established. Hyperglycaemia and hyperuricaemia occur. These adverse reactions and the occurrence of extrapyramidal signs during long-term oral treatment reduce its acceptability to patients.

Several other agents—old and new—are available as alternatives to the above drugs.

RAUWOLFIA DERIVATIVES

Many rauwolfia derivatives are available either alone (seven preparations) or in combination (14 preparations). Their effectiveness in lowering blood pressure is well established. Despite the number of preparations marketed, their popularity as first-choice treatment, alone or in combination with other drugs, is waning. Adverse reactions include mild sedation, increased dreaming, and occasionally adverse effects on mood, particularly in patients with a tendency towards depression. In addition, an association between rauwolfia derivatives and an increased incidence of breast cancer has been claimed, and disputed.

PRAZOSIN

Prazosin is an effective new hypotensive agent that acts directly on the relaxation of vascular smooth muscle. Side effects are predictable on the basis of a knowledge of the mode of action but some individual variations in response have been reported. In particular some patients have experienced a sudden loss of consciousness within 30 to 90 minutes of receiving the initial dose. It is now recommended that the initial dose should be of 0·5 mg or less, taken with food and late in the day because hypotension and syncope may occur if the initial dose is excessive. Prazosin is usually prescribed thrice daily up to a total daily dosage of 20 mg. Increments in doses should not be made at more than four- to six-week intervals.

Hypertension

GANGLION-BLOCKING AGENTS

Ganglion-blocking agents such as pentolinium are now seldom used.

PERSONAL POLICY

Mild hypertension

Older patients—My personal preference is a diuretic, usually bendrofluazide 5 mg once daily, with appropriate potassium supplements.

Younger patients (<65 *years*)—My first choice is a beta-blocker, usually propranolol (<320 mg/day) in two doses.

Moderate hypertension

I introduce the second agent (either thiazide or beta-blocker) after two to four weeks treatment with one drug alone. The next addition to the "cocktail" is hydrallazine (<100 mg/day) in younger patients, or methyldopa (<1500 mg/day) in older patients. I do not initiate treatment nowadays with adrenergic neurone blockers, clonidine, or reserpine.

CONCLUSION

The decision to start treatment and the choice of drug depends on a knowledge of patient and drug factors. Treatment should not be started on the basis of flimsy evidence of raised blood pressure. The reduction in blood pressure should not be associated with unacceptable adverse effects. In patients with severe hypertension, treatment with a combination of low doses of different agents may increase the compliance of the patient with long-term tablet taking. A dramatic reduction in blood pressure over the space of a few minutes is essential only in hypertensive crises, and the uncritical and overenthusiastic use of potent parenteral antihypertensive agents should be discouraged.

REFERENCES

1 Kannel, W B, and Dawber, T R, *British Journal of Hospital Medicine*, 1974, **11,** 508.
2 Veterans Administration Co-operative Study Group, *Journal of the American Medical Association*, 1967, **202,** 1028.
3 Veterans Administration Co-operative Study Group, *Journal of the American Medical Association*, 1970, **213,** 1143.
4 Veterans Administration Co-operative Study Group, *Circulation*, 1972, **45,** 991.
5 Taguchi, J, and Freis, E D, *New England Journal of Medicine*, 1974, **291,** 329.
6 American Heart Association Report, *Circulation*, 1967, **36,** 980.

Management of acute myocardial infarction

J F PANTRIDGE, J S GEDDES

Each year in Britain over 55 000 deaths among people under 70 result from myocardial infarction. Nearly two-thirds of these premature deaths are classified as sudden, as they occur within one hour of the onset of symptoms. Asystolic arrest usually related to acute atrioventricular block is responsible for a few deaths, but more than 90% of the sudden deaths from ischaemic heart disease result from ventricular fibrillation. Since the median delay in hospital admission may be more than eight hours, the hospital coronary care unit cannot influence the incidence of sudden death nor will it appreciably reduce the community mortality from the acute coronary attack, which is about 40%. Furthermore, the hospital coronary care unit will not affect the incidence of cardiogenic shock or pump failure, since these complications are manifestations of an extensive infarct. Clinical and experimental evidence indicates that after coronary occlusion there is often progressive increase in the amount of myocardium destroyed and the size of the infarct is determined in the first few hours. Early therapeutic intervention may limit the magnitude of the infarct.

Since the incidence of ventricular fibrillation is highest immediately after the onset of symptoms and since treatment to limit the size of the infarct and prevent shock and pump failure is likely to be most effective if started at the onset of the coronary episode, the early initiation of intensive care is clearly imperative.

VENTRICULAR FIBRILLATION

The correction of ventricular fibrillation outside hospital has been shown to be a practical proposition.[1 2] This has led to the development of mobile coronary care units, many of them staffed by medical personnel. It has been found, however, that paramedical workers are quite capable of correcting ventricular fibrillation. In the USA, in addition to mobile units, life-support stations have been installed in football stadia, skyscraper office blocks, factories, and airports. In Seattle about 25% of the adult population have been instructed in cardiopulmonary resuscitation. In that city (population 400 000) there were 73 long-term survivors among those defibrillated outside hospital by paramedical workers in one year. If this figure is applicable to the cities in Britain some 4000 lives might be saved annually by correcting ventricular fibrillation outside hospital.

The report of a working party of the Royal College of Physicians and British Cardiac Society on the care of the patient with coronary disease[3] stated that: "widespread instruction of the public in resuscitation should be encouraged as a further means of rescuing victims stricken by acute heart attacks. Such instruction could be carried out by trained laymen or medical personnel in schools, factories, and large institutions." Further involvement of the public has been suggested, and Friedberg has stated that "possibly every home with a person at risk should have a portable defibrillator next to the television set." In buildings occupied by many people, particularly middle-aged men, it might be appropriate to mount portable defibrillators beside the fire extinguishers. Furthermore, a portable defibrillator should be part of the equipment of general practitioners and doctors who are likely to encounter medical emergencies.

The major barriers to the widespread availability of portable defibrillators for use outside hospital relate to their cost, bulk, and weight. The claim of Tacker and co-workers that defibrillators should be capable of delivering more energy than they do at present is calculated to heighten the barriers. The view that high-energy direct-current shock is necessary, however, has been challenged and indeed a miniature defibrillator weighing 3·2 kg is available.[4 5]

Prevention

The prevention of ventricular fibrillation presents difficulties. In hospital coronary care units prophylactic antiarrhythmic agents are administered when R on T ectopics are evident or when ventricular ectopics are multifocal, occur in salvos, or occur more frequently than six a minute. This is not a rational policy during the acute phase since it is now recognised that about 40% of patients who develop ventricular fibrillation do so without prior warning dysrhythmias. Ideally, therefore, if an effective prophylactic antiarrhythmic agent were available it should be given to all patients when first seen. It has been claimed that lignocaine reduces the risk of ventricular fibrillation when given as an intravenous bolus of 100 mg followed immediately by an infusion of 3 mg/min. Nevertheless, lignocaine may be less effective during the acute phase than later in the attack. It may fail to control ventricular ectopics and may have an adverse effect when the heart rate is over 90 beats/min.

The high incidence of ventricular fibrillation immediately after the onset of acute infarction and the difficulty in its prevention at that time may relate to the frequency of the autonomic disturbance associated with coronary occlusion. Among patients seen within 30 minutes of the onset of the coronary attack over 80% show clinical evidence of autonomic disturbance.[5 6] Nearly half show evidence of parasympathetic overactivity, with bradycardia or hypotension, or both. More than one-third show sympathetic overactivity with tachycardia or transient hypertension, or both.

Treatment

Pain may accentuate or indeed initiate autonomic disturbance. Its relief is therefore of primary importance. Catecholamine release, which is significantly related to the development of ventricular dysrhythmias, may be diminished by the immediate control of pain. Analgesics used in relieving the pain of acute myocardial infarction should also relieve distress and fear. The ideal analgesic should have a rapid effect without causing nausea, vomiting, or haemodynamic deterioration.

Pethidine and pentazocine have potential adverse haemodynamic effects. Narcotic drugs are usually advocated despite their respiratory depressant effect.

Morphine is the drug most commonly used. Administered intravenously, 10 mg will usually relieve pain rapidly and alleviate mental distress. Heroin, however, is the narcotic drug of choice. It has a more rapid action and less emetic effect than morphine. When given in the standard intravenous dose of 5 mg it has little haemodynamic effect. After the administration of a narcotic drug hypotension may occur on tilting or during transport with the feet dependent. Every effort should therefore be made to keep the patient supine.

BRADYARRHYTHMIA

Sinus bradycardia requires treatment only when accompanied by hypotension or ventricular extrasystoles. Nevertheless, uncomplicated bradycardia in the acute phase of myocardial infarction is uncommon. Bradycardia immediately after the onset of acute infarction is usually associated with hypotension, which in most cases may be corrected by raising the heart rate. The slow heart rate is associated with a fall in ventricular fibrillation threshold and an increased risk of ventricular fibrillation. Conversely, raising the heart rate to normal may abolish ventricular ectopics and reduce the risk.

When atropine is required for correcting sinus bradycardia it is given intravenously in aliquots. Careful monitoring is mandatory during administration of the drug since an inappropriate and dangerous increase in the heart rate may result. Early atrioventricular block, second degree or complete, will usually respond to atropine. The dose required for the correction of atrioventricular block, however, is usually much larger than that required for treating sinus bradycardia.

TACHYCARDIA

The tachycardia associated with sympathetic overactivity lowers the ventricular fibrillation threshold. In the patient with recent coronary occlusion an increase in the heart rate occurring spontaneously or resulting from the injudicious administration of atropine may precipitate ventricular fibrillation. Antiarrhythmic agents may fail to control ventricular ectopics unless the tachycardia associated with sympathetic overactivity is corrected. An inappropriately rapid heart rate may occur during movement in more than one-third of patients with acute myocardial infarction. This may be relevant to the frequency of arrhythmic death in ambulances. Thus monitoring during transport is imperative.

Tachycardia resulting from sympathetic overactivity may be controlled by a beta-adrenergic blocking agent. It is doubtful whether the effects of the various non-selective beta-blocking agents differ appreciably when given in equivalent beta-blocking dosage. Sotalol, which does not possess intrinsic sympathomimetic activity, has been found effective in controlling tachycardia even when the rate is in excess of 120 beats/min. One or two aliquots of 5 mg are given intravenously and a decrease in heart rate is usually apparent within 2 minutes. Practolol, a selective cardiac beta-blocker with intrinsic sympathomimetic activity, has also been used. It has a less powerful negative chronotropic effect than sotalol, but it may be safer when intense bronchospasm is present.

PREVENTION OF SHOCK AND CARDIAC FAILURE

Since established cardiogenic shock is associated with massive infarction its treatment is seldom rewarding. Clinical studies[7 8] and recent experimental evidence, however, indicate that the magnitude of the infarct may be limited. After coronary occlusion irreversible damage begins within 20 minutes in totally ischaemic regions but survival is more prolonged in much of the affected zone. Many cells may recover provided the intensity of ischaemia does not increase. The fate of such jeopardised myocardium is determined by the balance of oxygen supply and demand. It has been rightly said that the quantity of jeopardised myocardium that can be salvaged varies inversely with the time after coronary occlusion that treatment begins. The loss of a critical amount of muscle may result from delay in treatment. This loss will further depress pump function. The resulting less favourable haemodynamic conditions jeopardise new areas and a vicious circle is begun.

That the incidence of shock may be reduced when haemodynamic disturbances secondary to autonomic imbalance are controlled early in the attack was shown in 1970.[7 8] Only 3·4% of patients aged 70 or less treated within one hour of the onset developed shock, with the result that the hospital mortality was under 10%. This may be contrasted with the prevailing mortality of 15–20% among patients treated in hospital coronary care units.

Blood flow to ischaemic myocardium through collateral vessels occurs mainly during diastole and is very sensitive to changes in arterial pressure. Hypotension and tachycardia therefore reduce flow. Oxygen requirement in contracting myocardium is also related to arterial pressure but to a lesser extent than blood flow. An increase in the blood pressure from hypotensive to normotensive levels may therefore have a favourable effect on myocardial survival. Oxygen requirement is also affected by the heart rate, the contractility of the myocardium, and the ventricular diastolic or filling pressure. A rise in the last, indicative of left ventricular failure, decreases blood flow by compressing the subendocardial zone. The associated dilatation of the left ventricle results in an increase in the work required to maintain the arterial pressure.

The early vagal overactivity of acute myocardial infarction is usually complicated by hypotension, which is often profound. Among patients seen within 30 minutes, 22% will have a systolic blood pressure not over 80 mm Hg.[6] Hypotension and resultant reduction in blood flow through ischaemic areas extend the boundaries of the developing infarct. Correction of early vagal overactivity and its associated bradycardia and hypotension with appropriate doses of atropine improves myocardial perfusion and prevents or limits extension of the infarct.

Sympathetic overactivity is associated with sinus tachycardia, with increased contractility, and not infrequently with transient hypertension. The resulting stress on the left ventricle may precipitate failure, which is often clinically unobtrusive. Reduced diastolic compliance (increased stiffness) of the ischaemic zone aggravates this effect. Thus sympathetic overactivity increases oxygen demand and curtails supply. Beta-adrenergic sympathetic blocking drugs control tachycardia and excessive contractility with little effect on ventricular filling pressure or arterial blood pressure (unless this is greatly increased). The longer diastolic intervals permit an increase in collateral flow. The viability of jeopardised cells is improved.

Hypotension in the absence of bradycardia and simulating cardiogenic shock is sometimes associated with inadequate venous return and a low ventricular filling pressure. When signs of left ventricular failure are absent 200 ml of a solution of 5% dextrose are infused rapidly, and if an increase in arterial pressure follows a volume expander such as low molecular weight dextran in 5% dextrose is infused for a few hours at a rate sufficient to maintain the systolic blood pressure at a level above 90 mm Hg.

Other therapeutic approaches directed towards limiting infarct size are at present the subject of intensive investigation.

Infusions of vasodilator drugs such as nitroglycerine and intravenous administration of frusemide effectively lower the ventricular filling pressure when this is raised, and provided the effects are monitored carefully a harmful reduction in blood pressure may usually be avoided. Bradycardia and hypotension occasionally develop and may be corrected with atropine. A reduction in S–T segment elevation after nitroglycerine in one clinical study suggested that ischaemia had been reduced.

Management of acute myocardial infarction

Myocardial oedema secondary to ischaemia increases vascular resistance and contributes to extension of the infarct. It may be reduced by administering mannitol, an osmotically active agent. The enzyme hyaluronidase may improve the transfer of substrates between the circulation and tissues, and a preliminary clinical trial of this agent has produced encouraging results. Glucose and glucose-insulin-potassium mixtures may provide metabolic support even in the absence of improved oxygenation. Corticosteroids when administered in high doses prevent the disruption of intracellular structures and may allow ischaemic tissues to survive until better haemodynamic conditions prevail.

Fortunately it is already possible to influence the incidence of shock by such simple measures as relieving pain and correcting the autonomic disturbance. It does not seem over-optimistic to expect that treatment begun soon after the onset of the attack with one or more of the recently introduced agents will further limit the size of the infarct.

PREHOSPITAL CORONARY CARE

Although most of the unnecessary deaths from acute myocardial infarction are sudden and occur outside hospital, and although most of the myocardial damage occurs in the first three hours, little attempt has been made in Britain to provide prehospital coronary care. The lack of enthusiasm for mobile coronary care units in this country despite their proliferation in the USA requires comment. Undoubtedly the concept of prehospital and hospital coronary care has been influenced adversely by the misunderstanding of the findings of the Bristol study. The report of the Bristol study[9] did not, of course, question the unassailable fact that most early deaths from acute myocardial infarction result from ventricular fibrillation, which may be corrected or prevented. Nor did that report question the fact that infarct size might be limited and cardiogenic shock and pump failure prevented.

The Bristol study purported to show that for some patients with myocardial infarction treatment at home might be satisfactory. This claim is not unrealistic. Intensive care has little to offer the patient who has survived the acute phase of the infarct. It is, however, salutary to consider the fate of patients in the Bristol study who sought medical advice within one hour but who presumably did not get intensive care at that time. The mortality was 26%. This is to be contrasted with a mortality of less than 10% in comparable patients who received intensive care within one hour of the onset of symptoms.[5 6]

It is unfortunate that prehospital coronary care schemes are assumed to be expensive in terms of personnel and equipment. The mobile coronary care unit may be integrated into the existing emergency system and the addition of a prehospital coronary care facility to the hospital coronary care unit should result in only a marginal increase in the cost, apart from that increase resulting from admitting those whose death outside hospital has been prevented. This latter cost may be diminished when attention is directed to the earlier discharge of patients no longer at risk. One-third of patients with acute myocardial infarction may be discharged on the third day.[10] When a higher proportion of patients get intensive care early, fewer will have large infarcts and, therefore, more will qualify for early discharge.

When the cost of prehospital coronary care is under consideration attention should be directed to the cost of the hospital coronary care unit and to the fact that in the absence of an associated prehospital coronary care scheme the hospital unit will have only a small impact on community mortality.[5 11] It is also salutary to remember the resources wasted in the unsuccessful treatment of cardiogenic shock. It is not unreasonable to suggest that much of the effort and expenditure directed to the treatment of shock by elaborate medical and surgical procedures might be redirected towards the prehospital phase and the prevention of these complications.

The report of the Working Party of the Royal College of Physicians of London and the British Cardiac Society[3] stated that "in view of the high death rate in the first three hours after an attack, the facilities that are generally available are inadequate. First, the public should be further instructed on the indications to call without delay upon emergency skilled help, and mobile coronary care units should be further developed. The exact means must depend on local conditions and requirements. Thus, their implementation should be on a local or regional basis, with the encouragement of the Department of Health and Social Security and the other national health authorities."

REFERENCES

1 Pantridge, J F, and Geddes, J S, *Lancet*, 1966, **1**, 807.
2 Pantridge, J F, and Geddes, J S, *Lancet*, 1967, **2**, 271.
3 Working Party of the Royal College of Physicians and the British Cardiac Society, *Journal of the Royal College of Physicians*, 1975, **10**, 5.
4 Pantridge, J F, *et al*, *British Medical Journal*, 1975, **2**, 313.
5 Pantridge, J F, *et al*, *The Acute Coronary Attack*. Tunbridge Wells, Pitman Medical, 1975.
6 Pantridge, J F, *et al*, in *Progress in Cardiology*, vol 3, ed P N Yu and J F Goodwin, p 173. Philadelphia, Lea and Febiger, 1974.
7 Pantridge, J F, *Quarterly Journal of Medicine*, 1970, **39**, 621.
8 Pantridge, J F, World Health Organisation, *Mobile Coronary Care Units*, EUR 5020. Copenhagen, WHO Regional Office for Europe, 1970.
9 Mather, H G, *et al*, *British Medical Journal*, 1971, **3**, 334.
10 Wilson, C, and Pantridge, J F, *Lancet*, 1973, **2**, 1284.
11 Pantridge, J F, *British Heart Journal*, 1974, **36**, 233.

Treatment of angina

DAVID SHORT

Nowhere is the aphorism "Diagnosis comes before treatment" more true than in managing angina pectoris.

Firstly, angina must be recognised. It is still often overlooked. Attacks of pain or oppression occurring anywhere in the torso (though usually in the region of the upper or middle sternum) precipitated by effort or emotion, and persisting for a few minutes, must be regarded as anginal. Radiation to one or both arms, the throat, lower jaw, or back provides further confirmation of the diagnosis. Difficulties in diagnosis arise when the pain is in an atypical site; dependent on a combination of exercise with cold or a recent meal; and induced by excitement rather than effort and the electrocardiogram is normal even when recorded during strenuous effort.

Secondly, it must be accepted that (malingering apart) a history of angina always indicates a reduced coronary reserve. It has often been claimed that hiatus hernia and other disorders of the oesophagus may produce an identical symptom, but this has never been proved.

Thirdly, it must be realised that a reduced coronary reserve does not necessarily imply narrowing of the coronary arteries, although that is by far the commonest cause. In perhaps 5% of cases angina may be due to other varieties of heart disease that cause either a reduction in coronary blood flow or an increase in myocardial work, or both—for instance, severe aortic valve disease, hypertension and, less commonly, cardiomyopathy, mitral stenosis, or pulmonary hypertension. Occasionally no evidence of heart disease (or any other disease) can be found.

Fourthly, it must be appreciated that even when angina is due basically to coronary arterial narrowing the symptom may be aggravated and the diagnosis complicated by extracardiac diseases. In the first place, there are diseases which decrease the oxygen content of the blood or increase the work of the heart—anaemia and thyrotoxicosis. Moreover, certain diseases—such as chronic cholecystitis, duodenal ulcer, or cervical spondylosis—may cause pain in the chest and aggravate and distort the pain of angina. Anxiety, smoking, and obesity are other aggravating factors that need to be considered in treating angina.

To treat angina rationally it is necessary not only to make a comprehensive diagnosis but also to appreciate the prognosis of different patterns of angina. Certain types of angina are particularly dangerous. Recent onset angina is in this category, especially if the onset is sudden. Crescendo angina—that is, angina increasing in severity without any extracardiac cause such as anaemia, increasing weight, or a fall in atmospheric temperature—also carries a high incidence of myocardial infarction and death. Angina that is unresponsive to adequate medical treatment also carries a serious prognosis. On the other hand, it is not sufficiently appreciated that in many patients angina subsides completely and may not return.

GENERAL PRINCIPLES OF TREATMENT

Any remediable factors such as severe aortic valve disease, mitral stenosis, hypertension, anaemia, thyrotoxicosis, as well as smoking and obesity, should be corrected. Gall bladder disease and duodenal ulceration should be treated, although operation should not as a rule be advised unless it is indicated on other grounds.

Patients with angina should be advised to avoid activities that bring on the pain. This usually means walking more slowly and avoiding exercise after a meal or in the coldest part of the day. They should be specifically warned against heavy lifting and pushing—for instance, lifting heavy furniture or trying to push a car which has become stuck. If they can avoid travelling to work in the rush-hour they should do so. It may be best to go earlier than usual when parking is easier. If the patient's occupation is strenuous and less heavy or demanding work is available a change should be advised; but unsuitable work is far better than unemployment. If the patient can move to a warm climate, this is to be recommended. There is some evidence to suggest that drugs such as the contraceptive pill and amitriptyline (Tryptizol) increase the risk of myocardial infarction and sudden death; such drugs should therefore be avoided so far as possible.

Nervous factors are very important in angina; indeed, Paul White went so far as to say that the nervous sensitivity of a patient was as important as all the pathological factors combined. For this reason an optimistic, reassuring attitude is important. Indeed, it is usually justified; for the prognosis of angina is nothing like as bad as it is often thought to be. Statements like, "You have a mild form of angina" and, "Your heart is 95% normal" are often appropriate. It is also important to avoid unnecessarily frequent review because frequent interrogation regarding symptoms tends to perpetuate them.

DRUG TREATMENT

Glyceryl trinitrate

Glyceryl trinitrate is still the mainstay of treatment and is usually sufficient in the mild case. The patient should be instructed to carry his tablets with him constantly in a container with a well-fitting cap (to avoid loss of potency by evaporation). He should be told to suck (not swallow) one of the tablets at the onset of pain or oppression. He should be advised to chew the tablet if the pain is severe and to discard it as soon as the symptom has been relieved. He should also be advised, until he is familiar with the effect of the tablet, to sit down after taking it, in order to minimise the danger of fainting. He should not be advised to lie down because this increases the work of the heart and tends to prolong the attack. It is also important to instruct the patient in the prophylactic use of the drug—that is, to suck a tablet before starting any exertion that he knows from experience is likely to bring on his angina.

Some patients find that glyceryl trinitrate in the standard dose of 0·5 mg causes such a headache that they prefer to put up with the angina. Such patients should be told that they are unusually sensitive to the preparation and need a smaller dose (0·3 mg) or, alternatively, that they should be advised to break the tablets and take half a tablet or less. The trinitrate may be replaced by a less rapid and longer-acting compound such as isosorbide dinitrate 5–20 mg three times a day. Other patients find glyceryl trinitrate tablets helpful but are afraid of over-using them for fear they will lose their efficacy or lead to harmful side effects. Such patients may be reassured on both accounts and told that as many as 20 tablets have been taken daily for long periods without harm.

There has been some concern about the loss of potency of trinitrate tablets. Earlier preparations using a cocoa base were somewhat unstable, but the modern tablets in a mannitol base retain their activity for at least two years if stored in an air-tight container, protected from light, and kept in a cool dry place. Heat accelerates decomposition, so that tablets kept in a waistcoat pocket might need to be changed rather sooner.

The way glyceryl trinitrate works is still not absolutely certain. Although a coronary vasodilator, the degree to which it can dilate zones of atherosclerotic narrowing is uncertain. It usually causes a rapid fall in blood pressure, which decreases the work of the heart. It also dilates the peripheral veins, with consequent pooling of blood in the hands and feet; this reduces the venous return to the heart, and hence its stroke output and work.

Beta-adrenergic blocking drugs

Propranolol (Inderal) and oxprenolol (Trasicor) were a great advance in treating patients with severe angina. Many new beta-blocking drugs have appeared in the last two or three years, but it is too early to say whether any has any advantage over the well-tried preparations. Practolol (Eraldin) should no longer be used for treating chronic angina on account of its occasional serious side effects. Not all patients are helped by beta-blockade: a few are actually made worse. Nevertheless, most patients improve and the results are often dramatic, particularly in patients with tachycardia or other evidence of sympathetic overactivity. In patients with associated hypertension beta-blockade offers a chance of "killing two birds with one stone."

It is wise to start treatment with a small dose—for example, propranolol 10 mg twice daily—and to double the dose every three or four days until relief is obtained, or the heart rate falls below 60 beats/min. If the angina remains unrelieved in spite of a reduction of heart rate below 60 beats/min, a larger dose may still be successful, but this should be done only with due caution. Care should be taken in patients with a tendency to bronchospasm, because this may be made worse. If there is cardiac enlargement beta-blockade should be accompanied by a diuretic (or digoxin), but if the resting electrocardiogram is normal this precaution is unnecessary. Since angina often subsides spontaneously it may not be necessary to continue beta-blockage indefinitely. If the patient is getting no angina at all the dose should be gradually reduced, and if the symptom does not return the drug may be stopped and kept in reserve.

Other drugs

With glyceryl trinitrate for the relief of the acute attack and beta-blocking drugs for continuous prophylaxis, the need for other drugs is greatly diminished. Nevertheless, there are patients who are not helped by beta-blockade and for whose frequent attacks of angina glyceryl trinitrate produces only transient relief. Many attempts have been made to find drugs with a more prolonged action than the nitrates, but without success. For patients with nocturnal angina one of the isosorbide dinitrate preparations is often valuable. Diazepam (Valium) may also be helpful, but stronger hypnotics have the disadvantage that they rarely abolish the attacks and often make the patient too confused to take his trinitrate properly. In such cases, a whisky nightcap may be effective. Perhexiline maleate (Pexid) has sometimes been dramatically successful in relieving angina that has been resistant to other treatment including beta-blockade. Verapamil hydrochloride (Cordilox) and prenylamine (Synadrin) have also been reported effective in some patients. The value of anticoagulant treatment and clofibrate (Atromid-S) now appears to be negligible.

SURGICAL TREATMENT

The operation of saphenous vein bypass, introduced five or six years ago, is a logical answer to what is basically a mechanical problem. The obstructed segment of a coronary artery is bypassed by a length of vein, whose proximal end is inserted into the aorta a short distance above the aortic valve and the distal end into the coronary artery beyond the obstruction. Two, three, or even four arteries may be grafted in this manner at one operation with very low mortality in experienced hands. Undoubtedly saphenous vein bypass is often dramatically successful in relieving severe angina that has proved resistant to full medical treatment including beta-blockade. On the other hand, there is no evidence yet that it alters the course of ischaemic heart disease or prolongs life. Hence it is quite unjustifiable at present to advocate this operation for all patients with angina.

Most patients with angina can live a more or less normal life with the help of glyceryl trinitrate and beta-blocking drugs, and a considerable proportion will lose their angina altogether. Others will develop myocardial infarction or die suddenly whatever is done. The only clear indication for saphenous vein bypass at present is angina that causes persistent disability after any remediable factors have been corrected and the medical armamentarium has been fully tried. Such patients should be seriously considered for operation, particularly if the electrocardiogram and *x*-ray films show only slight myocardial damage.

TREATMENT OF RECENT ONSET AND CRESCENDO ANGINA

Recent onset and crescendo angina, often referred to as unstable angina, carry a high risk of myocardial infarction or sudden death. If the angina appears only with effort, it is usually sufficient to insist on complete bodily and mental rest, reinforced by sedation if necessary. This often breaks the vicious circle, so that the patient may resume activity without the return of angina. If the attacks come on at rest as well as with effort it is clearly no use merely putting the patient to bed: more is required, though there is no agreement as to the best policy in such cases. If anxiety is a factor, as it often is, sedation is logical. If there is evidence of sympathetic overactivity one of the beta-blocking drugs is indicated. Anticoagulant treatment, either with heparin or warfarin, has its advocates, though it is by no means always successful in averting myocardial infarction. Thrombolytic treatment, using streptokinase, is currently being tried with some promising results. Saphenous vein bypass has also been tried in these cases, but the results to date are not encouraging.

Cardiac failure

JOHN HAMER

Although the prognosis of congestive cardiac failure remains serious, with an outlook as gloomy as that for many malignancies, there is no doubt that modern treatment, particularly the more potent diuretic drugs, has greatly improved the situation for many patients, who are kept alive and relatively comfortable on the "diuretic life" in a way which would not have been possible 20 years ago.

HEART RATE

The first question to consider in assessing a patient with congestive heart failure (using this term to include both pulmonary and systemic venous congestion) is: Is the heart rate appropriate? Either undue bradycardia or tachycardia may be a problem.

Bradycardia

Congestive heart failure in complete heart block may be improved by pacing, particularly in the elderly patient with heart block due to isolated disease of the conducting system, as the working myocardium is generally normal and effective control of the heart rate will help to relieve dyspnoea and oedema by control of the heart rate, restoring the patient to normal activities. Although Adams-Stokes attacks are the usual indication for pacing in complete heart block, congestive cardiac failure must not be overlooked as a possible presentation of complete heart block which is potentially remediable with modern treatment.

Tachycardia

Undue tachycardia is particularly seen as a factor producing congestive heart failure at the onset of atrial fibrillation. In a patient with a normal conducting system atrial fibrillation will produce a rapid and irregular ventricular rate. The duration of diastole is particularly affected by tachycardia as the time taken by each systole is reduced relatively little as the heart rate increases. Patients with mitral stenosis, one of the prime causes of atrial fibrillation, are particularly sensitive to the effects of tachycardia, as the shortening of diastole further impairs left ventricular filling which is obstructed by the mitral stenosis. A similar effect may be seen if ventricular filling is impaired by myocardial disease.

Pulmonary oedema at the onset of atrial fibrillation is characteristic of patients with severe mitral stenosis, and optimally mitral valvotomy should be carried out before such a critical complication can occur.

Cardiac failure

Control of the ventricular rate in atrial fibrillation and other atrial tachyarrhythmias is the prime indication for digitalis treatment, but the onset of the impairment of atrioventricular nodal conduction by vagal stimulation with digitalis is gradual even after intravenous administration, and a prompter response may be obtained by using an intravenous beta-adrenergic-blocking drug, particularly if there is no serious myocardial disturbance that might be adversely affected. Practolol, up to 10 mg intravenously, has the advantage of familiarity, and a single intravenous dose is not associated with the risks of eye changes and other complications found with long-term oral treatment. Prompt control of the ventricular rate in this way may be followed by long-term control with digitalis treatment. In atrial flutter near toxic doses of digitalis are needed to secure the 4:1 ventricular response associated with a satisfactory ventricular rate. A frequent experience is that 4:1 flutter at rest changes promptly to 2:1 flutter with troublesome tachycardia on exercise. This effect is due to the improvement in atrioventricular conduction produced by sympathetic stimulation on exercise. Advantage can be taken of the synergistic effect of digitalis and beta-adrenergic-blocking drugs on atrioventricular conduction to combine a modest dose of digitalis with beta-adrenergic blockade to eliminate the effect of sympathetic stimulation on exercise. In this way satisfactory control of the heart rate may be obtained without producing toxic effects from either group of drugs. Similar principles may be applied to controlling the ventricular rate in the occasional patient with atrial fibrillation showing an undue tachycardia on exercise, but care must be taken that the adverse effect of beta-adrenergic blockade on myocardial function does not produce a deterioration in congestive heart failure in patients with myocardial disease. The improvement in congestive heart failure recently reported in patients with myocardial disease following beta-adrenergic blockade[1] may be related to control of undue tachycardia in this particular group of patients with myocardial disease after acute myocarditis, but the problems of this treatment are so great that it should not be embarked on without expert advice.

Conversely, in other cases tachycardia may be part of the compensatory mechanism. The shortened diastole of tachycardia helps reduce the haemodynamic disturbance in severe aortic incompetence, and tachycardia is a major feature of the gross sudden aortic incompetence seen with destruction or perforation of the aortic valve in infective endocarditis. Under these circumstances too rigorous control of the tachycardia may have an adverse effect on the cardiac output. Tachycardia is a major factor maintaining the circulation if the stroke volume is much reduced as in pericardial tamponade, and it has even been suggested that isoprenaline should be used to increase the rate further as an emergency measure in these cases.

DIGITALIS TREATMENT

Although digitalis treatment has long been regarded as mandatory in congestive heart failure and is invaluable in the control of atrial fibrillation, considerable doubt has been expressed recently about its long-term beneficial effect in congestive heart failure in patients with sinus rhythm. Objective studies have failed to show sustained improvement,[2] and it may be that the diseased myocardium has a limited response and that any improvement in contractility produced by digitalis treatment leads to a reduction in myocardial drive by other compensatory mechanisms such as sympathetic nerve stimulation or the Frank-Starling effect. The prime indication for digitalis treatment remains the control of the ventricular rate in atrial fibrillation and in this role it is effective and convenient.

Probably much digitalis toxicity has arisen from the inappropriate search for a beneficial effect of digitalis on myocardial contractility in patients with congestive heart failure in normal sinus rhythm. In atrial fibrillation the control of the ventricular rate provides a useful and convenient index of digitalis effect. The ventricular rate should be measured, as in the early stages of treatment the rapid and irregular ventricular rate may not be transmitted consistently to the peripheral pulse. With increasing atrioventricular block during digitalis treatment the ventricular rate becomes slower and less irregular and the difference between the ventricular and peripheral pulse rate is reduced. Nevertheless, ventricular ectopic beats produced as a toxic effect of digitalis treatment may not be transmitted to the peripheral pulse, and alternating ventricular ectopic beats may produce an apparent halving of the effective heart rate. The useful rule that a dose should be omitted if the heart rate falls below 60/min has saved many patients from digitalis poisoning. Digitalis overdosage is to be suspected if the heart rate becomes completely regular—a slow regular rate suggesting complete heart block with a junctional (atrioventricular nodal) escape rhythm, a more rapid regular rate the onset of atrial tachycardia with a regular, say 2:1, ventricular response. In patients with sinus rhythm the useful changes in heart rate found with digitalis treatment in atrial fibrillation are not evident; the tendency to slowing expected on pharmacological grounds may be obscured by other effects on the heart rate in patients with congestive heart failure and cannot be expected to give a guide to the control of digitalis treatment. Digitalis must therefore be used with great caution in patients with sinus rhythm. The risk of toxicity from digitalis glycosides is so great that they should not be pushed to obtain a probably illusory beneficial effect on contractility in patients with congestive heart failure in sinus rhythm.

Cardiac failure

Digoxin

The availability of a plasma radioimmunoassay for digoxin favours the use of digoxin rather than the other digitalis glycosides, for which little advantage can be shown. The recent problems of variation in biological availability with different preparations of digoxin tablet have been overcome, and all British tablets now have a uniform standard of high availability. Digoxin is primarily handled by renal excretion and maintenance doses must be correspondingly reduced in the presence of renal failure. This policy seems preferable to using a different glycoside in patients with renal disease such as digitoxin, which is handled by hepatic excretion. Suggestions that particular glycosides are less likely to cause nausea and vomiting are unsupported by objective data, and there is little evidence that any of the purified glycosides are preferable in this respect. Although nausea may not be the earliest sign of toxicity, in that arrhythmias may occur without nausea, it should be regarded as suggestive of excessive treatment. Antiemetic drugs should never be given to allow continuation of the dose of digitalis that produces nausea.

A loading dose of digoxin is necessary to start treatment but the onset of action is gradual even after absorption so there is little advantage from parenteral administration; if quick control of heart rate is needed it is better to use an alternative treatment such as an intravenous beta-adrenergic-blocking drug or electroversion (DC shock). Some of the most exciting examples of digitalis poisoning are seen when a loading dose of a digitalis glycoside is given to a patient who is receiving a maintenance dose of digitalis prescribed elsewhere. Careful inquiry must be made before prescribing, remembering that an unfamiliar preparation may be in use, particularly in patients treated abroad. If there is any doubt and treatment is not urgent a standard maintenance dose of digoxin will be effective in a few days. A loading dose of digoxin in an average sized man might be 1 mg followed by 0·5 mg twice daily for one day and a maintenance dose of 0·25 mg twice daily with further adjustment according to the response after a few days. Some patients seem to have problems of absorption even with tablets of known high availability and may need unexpectedly large doses. Patients with severe heart disease tend to need small doses, perhaps because of impaired renal function and may be maintained on as little as 0·0628 mg daily. This small tablet is also useful in treating patients needing smaller doses than usual; these include patients with renal disease and the elderly, probably because of reduced renal function, patients of small body build, and those with hypokalaemia. Although the potentiation of digitalis effect by hypokalaemia has been questioned,[3] there is good evidence[4] that the effect is a real one, as expected on theoretical grounds, although a definitive study is awaited.

Hypokalaemia

Hypokalaemia is particularly troublesome in patients with congestive heart failure as it may complicate concurrent diuretic treatment. The observation of a patient developing digitalis toxicity without change in digitalis dose when a diuretic is added to the regimen may be due to hypokalaemia or to impaired renal function as a result of diuretic treatment. Every effort should be made to avoid hypokalaemia from diuretic treatment in patients who are also being treated with digitalis glycosides.

Thyroid disease

The variation in response to digitalis treatment in patients with thyroid disease is probably at least in part related to changes in renal function; the patient with myxoedema being particularly sensitive to digoxin, and conversely, unexpectedly large doses being needed in thyrotoxicosis. The finding of similar changes in sensitivity to other glycosides, such as digitoxin, which are not excreted in the kidney suggests that variations in tissue sensitivity with changes in thyroid function also play a part.

Digitalis toxicity

Digitalis toxicity usually presents as a rhythm disturbance, although nausea and vomiting may precede or accompany the rhythm change. Coloured vision, though not infrequent if sought with special tests, is rarely a cause of complaint. Intestinal disturbances with ulceration in the small intestine occur, particularly in the elderly. Ectopic atrial or ventricular tachyarrhythmias or atrioventricular block may occur, and the combination of tachycardia and block as in atrial tachycardia with a 2:1 or an irregular ventricular response is particularly characteristic. Apparent failure to control atrial fibrillation with a persisting rapid irregular rhythm may be due to a toxic atrial tachycardia with an irregular ventrical response. Occasional ventricular ectopic beats may accompany apparently satisfactory control of atrial fibrillation but are evidence that toxic levels are being approached, but regular alternating ventricular ectopic beats (bigeminy) should not be tolerated. Plasma digoxin levels taken at the steady state (at least four and preferably six hours after an oral dose) are useful in controlling treatment but cannot give an absolute guide because of other factors such as the plasma potassium concentration and probable thyroid state that influence the effectiveness of digitalis treatment. A steady-state plasma digoxin between 1·3 and 2·6 nmol/l (1 and 2 ng/ml) is usually satisfactory. A concentration below 1·3 nmol/l generally indicates ineffective treatment, but some patients with atrial fibrillation have natural disease of the atrioventricular conduction system that may prevent a rapid ventricular rate even without digitalis treatment. Most patients with satisfactory control of atrial fibrillation have steady-state plasma digoxin concentrations between 1·3 and 2·6 nmol/l. Levels above 2·6 nmol/l indicate a risk of toxic effects. Patients being treated with other glycosides, however, may show some response to a digoxin radioimmunoassay, although this will not reflect the true effect of treatment. Radioimmunoassays for other glycosides are not generally available and there is some advantage in the complementary assay techniques based on the action of digitalis glycosides on the Na and K dependent ATPase of the red cell that is responsive to all the glycosides in a manner corresponding to their cardiac effect; this method is not as well understood or as freely available as the digoxin radioimmunoassay.

In treating digitalis toxicity, stop the drug and correct any hypokalaemia. It may be worth while to withhold potassium-depleting diuretics until the condition is under control, when the whole regimen may be reconsidered to avoid any recurrence. Atrial tachyarrhythmias rarely need specific treatment but ventricular tachyarrhythmias are dangerous, as fatal ventricular fibrillation may follow. Multiform ventricular ectopic beats are a serious warning sign. Electroversion (DC shock) must be avoided in the presence of excess digitalis, as the digitalis effect is potentiated after the shock and may produce ventricular fibrillation or heart block. If such treatment is essential, as in cardiac arrest from ventricular fibrillation, the smallest possible energy of shock should be used. Beta-adrenergic-blocking drugs should not be used, as control of the tachyarrhythmia may be associated with potentiation of the digitalis effect on atrioventricular conduction, leading to complete heart block with suppression of the usual escape pacemakers by the beta-adrenergic blockade. It is better to suppress the ventricular ectopic rhythms with a drug such as lignocaine, which has little effect on atrioventricular conduction, or phenytoin sodium (Epanutin), which has a positively beneficial effect, improving atrioventricular conduction but is difficult to handle because of its unusual pharmacokinetic properties (very large loading dose and saturation kinetics). Lignocaine as used in cardiac infarction, an initial bolus of 100 mg followed by a continuous infusion at 1 to 2 mg/min, is generally satisfactory and should be the first choice as the most familiar treatment.

GENERAL MEASURES

Bed rest is useful in allowing the best use of a limited cardiac output and avoiding the effects of exercise in diverting blood flow to skeletal muscles, myocardium, and skin (for heat loss) at the expense of the visceral and, most significantly, the renal blood flow. It is common experience that admission to hospital leads to improvement in congestive failure without change in drug treatment. Sunbathing is occasionally possible, even in Britain, and should be avoided as it produces an obligatory cutaneous vasodilatation that diverts blood from more important vascular beds. In tropical conditions air conditioning is an advantage. If there is gross oedema or prolonged bed rest is thought likely to be needed prophylactic anticoagulant treatment should be started, as venous thrombosis and pulmonary embolism are common complications of congestive heart failure that may interfere with an otherwise satisfactory response to treatment.

DIURETIC TREATMENT

The mainstay of current management of congestive heart failure, diuretic treatment, does not improve cardiac function but removes troublesome oedema, which relieves symptoms such as breathlessness and allows greater activity, although there is good evidence that cardiac output falls further rather than improves with this treatment.[5]

Modern diuretics are generally so potent in removing excess sodium from the body that there is little need for a low-salt diet provided excessively salty foods such as kippers and bacon are avoided and additional salt is not added to the food. The excess of water in the body is generally secondary to sodium retention and limitation of water intake is not needed except in special circumstances (see below). Mercurial diuretics are now of historical interest only as their toxicity limited administration to twice a week. Carbonic anhydrase inhibitors had a brief vogue, but are relatively weak diuretics and tolerance develops quickly, so they are not important except as preliminaries to the development of the thiazide diuretics.

Thiazide diuretics are the mainstay of current treatment. Duration of action is the only real difference between the various analogues, and relative potency is of little importance as larger doses of the less potent agents may be given without toxic effects. Other moderately potent non-thiazide diuretics seem to offer little advantage. These drugs are often combined in tablet form with a modest dose of a potassium supplement, which can only be beneficial in helping to prevent potassium depletion secondary to the sodium diuresis, provided it does not obscure the fact that the dose of potassium provided may be grossly inadequate as a replacement treatment in an intensive diuretic regimen. As Slow-K is such a satisfactory potassium supplement I generally use the corresponding thiazide diuretic cyclopenthiazide (0·25 mg) with potassium (Navidrex-K). In mild congestive heart failure 0·25 mg twice daily will generally prove effective in maintenance treatment. A bed-time dose may produce troublesome diuresis during the night and it is usual to give the second dose of the day after lunch, but there is little difference in effect if the whole dose is given in the morning. It has been suggested that treatment on alternate days will avoid potassium depletion by allowing the body to correct the potassium loss on the day off treatment, but the alternate-day treatment produces a return of congestion on the day off treatment, which may be inconvenient, and in all but the mildest cases daily treatment is needed for effective control.

Loop diuretics—The newer agents such as frusemide, ethacrynic acid, and bumetanide have a more potent effect on sodium transport in the renal tubules than the thiazides and as they are relatively free of toxic effects have allowed control of more severe degrees of congestive heart failure. My experience is mainly with frusemide, which is given in very large doses (1 g intravenously) without toxic effect in renal failure. Although the previously untreated patient may be sensitive to relatively small doses, the usual maintenance regimen is 40 mg twice a day by mouth. A single dose of 80 mg each morning seems just as effective as divided doses. The response is relatively rapid and divided doses with the second dose on return from work may avoid nocturnal breathlessness without a noticeable diuresis during the night. In general the diuretic dose needed to eliminate oedema and reach dry weight in hospital is similar to the dose needed to maintain the position when the patient increases his activity on return home and the temptation to try to wean the patient off diuretics when free of oedema must be resisted. Excessive, inappropriate treatment, however, may produce a salt-depleted state.

POTASSIUM DEPLETION

The increase in sodium load reaching the distal renal tubules with diuretic treatment increases the activity of the sodium-potassium exchange system of the distal tubules that is under the control of aldosterone, and potassium and hydrogen ions are lost in exchange for retained sodium ions. Potassium depletion is a major feature of the patient with treated congestive heart failure held at dry weight by intensive diuretic treatment[6] and the condition is accentuated by hyperaldosteronism.[7] The potassium depletion may be partly evident as a fall in plasma potassium concentration, but the true depletion shown by measuring total body potassium is generally much greater than expected on the basis of plasma measurements. Much of the depletion is due to reduction in lean body mass, evident as the wasting of cardiac cachexia and there is little evidence of a reduced concentration of potassium in the cells.[10 11] The plasma potassium concentration is important as it may be reflected in symptoms such as fatigue or lethargy and is associated with potentiation of a digitalis effect that may lead to toxicity if digitalis treatment is being given concurrently with diuretics, as is often the case. Fortunately the plasma potassium seems to form part of a labile potassium pool, which is easily corrected by giving potassium supplements.[10 11] An increase in oral potassium intake can compensate for the renal potassium loss sufficiently to maintain a normal plasma potassium concentration. In Britain an attempt to increase potassium intake by changes in diet is generally unsatisfactory as unacceptable and too expensive, although instant coffee and fruit juice, but not squash, are good sources, and it is usual to give potassium supplements. In view of the associated alkalosis potassium should be given as the chloride rather than the bicarbonate, and local ulceration where the tablet dissolves has been overcome by using slow-release preparations such as Slow-K. Two tablets three times a day are generally satisfactory, but care must be taken that deteriorating renal function does not interfere with potassium excretion and lead to dangerous hyperkalaemia, so regular measurements of plasma electrolytes are a worthwhile precaution.

ALDOSTERONE ANTAGONISTS

An alternative policy is to block or reverse the distal tubular sodium-potassium exchange with drugs that oppose the action of aldosterone. Nicholls *et al*[7] have shown that there is a modest increase in plasma aldosterone in untreated congestive heart failure, a fall to low levels during diuresis, probably as renin secretion is reduced by the high sodium load in the distal tubules, followed by a rise of plasma aldosterone to very high levels as the patient approaches dry weight. The use of aldosterone antagonists has the advantage over potassium supplements that more of the less labile cellular potassium pool[10 11] may be replaced, and loss of other ions such as hydrogen ions and more subtle and less well-studied factors such as loss of magnesium ions may also be reversed, although it seems unlikely that the depleted cellular potassium can be completely restored unless the underlying heart disease can be cured, as by surgical correction of severe valve disease. A case can be made for using aldosterone antagonists in all stages of congestive heart failure because although plasma aldosterone is low during diuresis the exchange mechanism is particularly active then as a large sodium load is reaching the distal tubule.

Two main groups of aldosterone antagonists are available—the specific antagonists such as spironolactone, which is structurally analogous to aldosterone and acts as a competitive antagonist; and structurally dissimilar agents such as triamterene and amiloride, which produce opposite effects to those of aldosterone in the distal renal tubule without specific antagonism. With all potassium-retaining diuretics there is a danger of hyperkalaemia if renal function is impaired and potassium supplements should not generally be given in addition to these drugs. Spironolactone (Aldactone) has a moderately effective gradual diuretic action and has been suggested as a possible sole diuretic treatment for moderately severe congestive heart failure. It is more often used in doses of 25 to 50 mg two or three times a day to prevent potassium depletion during treatment with other diuretics.

Amiloride (Midamor), which has largely replaced the similar but less effective triamterene (Dytac), is not a specific aldosterone antagonist, although this may be an advantage in the severe hyperaldosteronism of the dried-out patient being maintained at dry weight by continued diuretic treatment in which very large doses of spironolactone would be needed to overcome the aldosterone effect, and the contrary action of amiloride may still be effective in spite of the high plasma aldosterone levels. Used in combination with frusemide at a ratio of 5 mg of amiloride with 40 mg of frusemide, amiloride generally maintains a normal plasma potassium concentration and removes the need for potassium supplements.

OTHER COMPLICATIONS OF DIURETIC TREATMENT

Sodium depletion

The sodium-retaining tendency in congestive heart failure is so potent that there is generally little risk of producing sodium depletion if diuretic treatment is tailored to the elimination of dyspnoea and troublesome oedema. Continued observation is needed as inappropriate excessive treatment may produce a salt-depleted state with haemoconcentration and gives a powerful stimulus to renin secretion and hyperaldosteronism. A very dramatic diuresis, as produced by a moderate intravenous dose of frusemide in a previously untreated patient, may produce a sharp reduction in circulating blood volume before oedema fluid can be mobilised to replace the loss. A similar shock-like state is well known after excessive venesection or the mechanical removal of ascites or the drainage of dependent oedema by acupuncture; these procedures are rarely needed nowadays as excess fluid can generally be removed gradually with diuretic treatment.

It may be injudicious to push diuretic treatment to restore venous pressures to normal in all circumstances as a raised venous pressure may be necessary for effective ventricular filling in some conditions. The large systolic wave in the jugular venous pulse from functional tricuspid incompetence can often be eliminated as the blood volume is reduced and the right ventricle becomes smaller, but a large venous "a" wave in the stiff right ventricle of severe pulmonary stenosis may play a vital part in right ventricular filling and should not be abolished. The similar situation in the left ventricle in severe aortic stenosis is less evident clinically but may account for some deterioration in left ventricle performance with intensive diuretic treatment. In constrictive pericarditis the high venous pressure is essential to fill the heart in the high-tension pericardial sac and should not be abolished. Treatment should not be increased after the elimination of troublesome oedema.

The dried-out patient with congestive heart failure exchanges the inconvenience and dangers of systemic and pulmonary oedema for a persistent low cardiac output state producing fatigue with hyperaldosteronism and the severe metabolic disturbance of cardiac cachexia. Treatment of congestive heart failure is not in any way curative and can be ragarded only as a palliative regimen that can keep the patient alive and may allow definitive surgical correction of the underlying disturbance if possible. Many units at any one time will have a few patients for whom cardiac transplantation seems the only feasible long-term answer.

Water retention

Not to be confused with sodium depletion, in which the plasma sodium remains normal but the extracellular blood volume is reduced, is hyponatraemia in congestive heart failure, which may occur in the dried-out state or be associated with persistent oedema. There is little evidence to support the suggestion that an excessive antidiuretic hormone effect is responsible. It seems more likely that a failure of free water clearance in the kidney results when the sodium load reaching the distal tubule is much reduced. There is a temptation to give sodium to improve the low plasma sodium concentration, but total body sodium is often increased in these patients as the extracellular fluid remains expanded. A response to administration of salt is reported at times, presumably as the sodium load to the distal tubules is transiently increased, but this treatment runs the risk of producing fatal pulmonary oedema. A better approach is to reduce water intake to daily losses plus 500 ml unless climatic conditions are extreme and continue conventional diuretic treatment. This regimen often provokes intense thirst, and it may be necessary to remove flower vases and other sources of temptation. An osmotic diuretic such as intravenous mannitol combined with intravenous frusemide to prevent any immediate increase in circulating plasma volume will often produce a water diuresis. In general hyponatraemia may be regarded as a terminal event, and if surgical treatment is considered feasible it may be justified to remove the excess water by dialysis, although the risk of any operation in those patients is very great.

PULMONARY OEDEMA

Left ventricular failure may present as dyspnoea on exertion or as paroxysmal nocturnal attacks, leading eventually to frank pulmonary oedema. Similar changes may occur in pulmonary congestion due to mechanical obstruction to left ventricular filling as in mitral stenosis. Radiological evidence of pulmonary congestion with distended upper-lobe veins, interstitial pulmonary oedema producing the horizontal

Kerley B lines at the costophrenic angles, and perihilar oedema may precede other clinical evidence of pulmonary congestion. Wheeziness from bronchial mucosal oedema is often a major feature, leading to the description as "cardiac asthma," probably because the bronchial veins communicate with the pulmonary veins and become congested as the pulmonary venous pressure rises. Wheeziness may cause diagnostic confusion with obstructive airways disease, particularly if both airways obstruction and left ventricular disease coexist, as is often the case in elderly patients in Britain. As some treatments recommended for left ventricular failure may be dangerous in airways obstruction it is useful to have a therapeutic programme suitable for use if the diagnosis is in doubt.

Morphine is the first line of treatment for left ventricular failure if the diagnosis is certain. It relieves dyspnoea by reducing the sensitivity of the respiratory centre to reflex stimulation from the stiff congested lung, reduces associated anxiety, and probably helps to shift fluid from the pulmonary to the systemic venous system by dilating systemic veins.

Aminophylline—In airways obstruction morphine might be fatal by reducing the sensitivity of the respiratory centre and critically impairing ventilation; a useful alternative is aminophylline 250 mg intravenously or 500 mg intramuscularly, which has a dramatic effect in relieving airways obstruction as well as a potent action in increasing myocardial contractility. In less acute situations aminophylline suppositories are useful and two at night may prevent paroxysmal nocturnal dyspnoea in the early hours of the morning. The treatment produces rectal irritation after a few nights but it is useful while other measures are becoming effective.

Salbutamol—Sympathomimetic drugs help relieve airways obstruction, but isoprenaline may have an adverse effect on the diseased heart, producing undesirable tachycardia or ventricular ectopic rhythms, and it is preferable to use the more selective agent salbutamol (Ventolin), which has little cardiac effect, particularly if given by inhalation.

Oxygen treatment—The presence of central cyanosis in left ventricular failure indicates a possible improvement from increasing the oxygen content of the inspired air. The relatively minor interference with gas transfer across the alveolar capillary membrane in pulmonary oedema is overcome sufficiently by hyperventilation to prevent a rise in arterial carbon dioxide tension and the arterial hypoxia is chiefly due to ventilation-perfusion imbalance with perfusion of underventilated alveoli. In left ventricular failure there is no contraindication to producing as high a concentration of inspired oxygen as possible, although in obstructive airways disease inspired oxygen is usually limited to avoid the complete removal of hypoxic ventilatory drive. In cases of doubt the use of a moderate increase in inspired oxygen is still of some beneficial effect. The Ventimask or similar system supplying a controlled mixture of inspired oxygen and ambient air is generally available for use in respiratory failure. Nasal catheters with a moderate flow of oxygen to avoid drying of the nasal mucosa similarly present a less controlled mixture of inspired oxygen and ambient air. It is in fact difficult to provide 100% oxygen unless the patient is being mechanically ventilated via an endotracheal tube and such a system produces a risk of pulmonary oxygen toxicity, one of the causes of "pump lung" after cardiopulmonary bypass. Other systems to supply 100% oxygen need a close-fitting mouth and nose piece with an oxygen reservoir to draw on during inspiration. In practice a moderate increase in inspired oxygen concentration is the best that can be achieved.

Pulmonary oedema is removed by diuretics as effectively as systemic oedema; this obvious treatment is sometimes overlooked as the oedema is not visible. In fact, removal of relatively small amounts of oedema from the lungs has a dramatic effect on symptoms. Intravenous frusemide will produce a dramatic response, but in a previously untreated patient the dose is much smaller than the usual oral doses for maintenance treatment and 10 mg intravenously is usually adequate. It is said that the diuresis begins before the needle can be withdrawn from the vein. An immediate local effect from dilatation of pulmonary veins is suspected. In older men with prostatic problems caution is needed with diuretic treatment as acute retention may be provoked. A preliminary rectal examination, easily carried out in the sitting position, is worth while.

Digitalis treatment—In acute left ventricular failure there may be transient beneficial effects from digitalis treatment, and digoxin 1 mg by mouth in a patient of normal build with no undue sensitivity is useful for starting treatment. If the situation is urgent half the initial dose may be given intravenously although the slow onset of action of digitalis glycosides after absorption reduces the advantages of intravenous treatment. The more rapidly acting glycoside medigoxin (Lanitop) may be useful here. In pulmonary oedema secondary to the rapid ventricular rate associated with the onset of atrial fibrillation as may be seen in mitral stenosis, control of the tachycardia has first priority, and the rapid action of beta-adrenergic-blocking drugs may be preferred to the more gradual action of digitalis glycosides.

Mechanical measures—The presence of a pleural effusion may critically increase dyspnoea in the patient with left ventricular failure. Effusion may arise in isolated left ventricular failure by transudation from the congested lung or secondarily to pulmonary infarction from venous thrombosis and embolism. Aspiration of a large pleural effusion may produce striking relief of breathlessness.

Venesection is a time-honoured treatment that may be appropriate if the jugular venous pressure is raised and has the effect of transferring blood from the pulmonary to the systemic venous system. Removal of too much blood too quickly may critically reduce ventricular filling. Removal of one pint (half a litre) is usually satisfactory, conventional blood donor equipment may be used, and the blood is usually suitable for transfusion. A similar effect can be produced less traumatically by venous occlusion with blood-pressure cuffs on the limbs.

Intermittent positive-pressure ventilation—Some patients with pulmonary oedema remain resistant to all these treatments. Attempts to remove froth from the airways by inhaling agents reducing surface tension have relatively little value in the pulmonary oedema of congestive heart failure, and in the intractable patient the best solution is endotracheal intubation which facilitates cleaning the airways followed by intermittent positive-pressure ventilation. The response is not due to forcing the oedema fluid back across the alveolar-capillary membrane but to the rise in intrathoracic pressure, which tends to keep blood in the systemic venous system and reduce the volume of blood in the pulmonary veins. In patients with mitral stenosis the induction of anaesthesia for mitral valvotomy may improve pulmonary oedema in a similar way.

Acute left ventricular failure carries serious prognostic implications. In hypertension it is a prime indication for effective control of blood pressure, and, although left ventricular failure *can* be controlled by antihypertensive drugs alone in these patients, this is a therapeutic tour de force which need not be repeated. Diagnostic confusion is sometimes produced by the transient rise of blood pressure that often accompanies the vasoconstrictor response to left ventricular failure in myocardial disease. In aortic stenosis one attack of left ventricular failure is an indication to consider aortic valve replacement as the natural history of aortic stenosis is such that further episodes of left ventricular failure are likely even with intensive treatment and each attack is progressively more difficult to treat. The tragedy of "death on the waiting list" is avoided only by prompt referral for operation after the first episode of left ventricular failure.

REFERENCES

[1] Waagstein, F, *et al*, *British Heart Journal*, 1975, **37**, 1022.
[2] Cohn, K, *et al*, *American Journal of Cardiology*, 1975, **35**, 461.
[3] Binnion, P F, *Lancet*, 1975, **1**, 343, 743.
[4] Shapiro, W, and Taubert, K, *Lancet*, 1975, **2**, 604.
[5] Stampfer, M, *et al*, *Circulation*, 1968, **37**, 900.
[6] White, R J, *et al*, *British Medical Journal*, 1969, **2**, 606.
[7] Nicholls, M G, *et al*, *Clinical Science and Molecular Medicine*, 1974, **47**, 301.
[8] Lawson, D H, *et al*, *Quarterly Journal of Medicine*, 1976, **45**, 469.
[9] Davidson, C, *et al*, *Lancet*, 1976, **2**, 1044.
[10] Nagent de Deuxchaisnes, C, *et al*, *Lancet*, 1961, **1**, 61.
[11] Nagent de Deuxchaisnes, C, and Mach, R S, *Lancet*, 1974, **1**, 517.

Diseases of the alimentary system

Absorption, distribution, and metabolism of drugs; effects of disease of the gut

C F GEORGE

Because the pharmacological and therapeutic effects of drugs are usually related to their free concentration in extracellular fluid a knowledge of the factors governing absorption, distribution, and eliminaton is essential to rational prescribing. Since most drugs are given by mouth, both for the convenience of the patient and because of the wide margin of safety that this route affords, the initial section of this article is confined to factors affecting absorption from the gut. It should, however, be remembered that advantages may result from a failure of drugs to be absorbed—for example, topical treatment with sulphonamides and corticosteroids may reduce the systemic side effects of these drugs in inflammatory disorders of the bowel.

DRUG ABSORPTION

The most important factors influencing absorption of drugs from the gastrointestinal tract are formulation, gastric and intestinal motility, physicochemical characteristics of the drug, and the surface area available for absorption.

Formulation

Drugs may be given by mouth in solution or suspension or as tablets, capsules, and slow-release preparations. Optimal absorption, however, cannot occur unless drugs are in solution by the time they reach the small intestine. Thus formulation is a major factor determining the rate and extent of absorption. An average tablet is a complex product with 20 or so constituents distributed between the core and its coating mass; typical ingredients include binding agents, diluents, disintegrating agents, dyes, and lubricants. Although various marketed brands of a single drug contain an identical amount, as dictated by the *British Pharmaceutical Codex*, and disintegrate in vitro within a specified time, they may differ in their rates of dissolution and particle size. Such variation between formulations may lead to major differences in the total amount of drug reaching the systemic circulation unchanged (bioavailability), as has been shown for digoxin, chloramphenicol, nitrofurantoin, phenindione, phenytoin, phenylbutazone, tolbutamide, and tetracyclines.[1]

Gastric and intestinal motility

A second major factor governing drug absorption is gastric emptying, which occurs exponentially at a rate that varies widely among individuals. For patients in whom gastric emptying is rapid, comparatively much of the dose is presented to the small intestine in a short time. If the formulation has ensured rapid dissolution in the stomach, drug absorption from the intestine can be both rapid and relatively complete. If, however, dissolution is slow but gastric emptying is rapid, undissolved drug will be presented to the small intestine and absorption may be incomplete—for example, certain brands of digoxin before September 1975. Gastric emptying may be modified by drug treatment and by surgery; metoclopramide improves the co-ordination of gastric muscular activity and thereby accelerates the rate of emptying, whereas anticholinergics (including many tricyclic antidepressants) have the opposite effect. The pattern and rate of gastric emptying may also be altered by partial gastrectomy or vagotomy and antrectomy. Drugs whose absorption has been shown to depend on gastric emptying include digoxin, levodopa, lithium carbonate, and paracetamol.

Intestinal motility is important in the absorption of water and electrolytes[2] but it also determines the time and surface area available for drug absorption.

Physicochemical characteristics

Physicochemical characteristics that are important in determining the absorption of drugs include the size of the molecule, its ionisation constant, and the lipid partition coefficient.

Most drugs used in clinical practice are of relatively low molecular weight: cholestyramine, a resin, is an exception and hence is unabsorbed. It can therefore be used to bind drugs within the gastrointestinal tract—for example, digitoxin—and will prevent enterohepatic recirculation of the latter. It also binds to warfarin and antibiotics[3] and reduces their absorption.

Many drugs are either weak acids or bases; hence they exist in both ionised and non-ionised forms. The extent of ionisation is determined by the ionisation constant, or pKa, which is defined as the pH at which half of a drug is in the ionised state. The importance of this concept is that a non-ionised drug is lipid-soluble and diffuses freely across cell membranes, whereas the ionised (charged) moiety cannot cross cell membranes. Thus in the case of aspirin, which has a pKa of 3·5, most of the drug is non-ionised in the stomach (pH 1–2), and much of it is absorbed from this organ. The absorption of aspirin is, however, diminished in pernicious anaemia.

Most basic drugs are absorbed from the small intestine, but even here only a small proportion of quaternary ammonium compounds are in the non-ionised state, and their absorption is poor. Certain highly charged chemicals including the herbicide paraquat may be actively absorbed by a carrier-mediated transport system. Once dissolved, however, the most important factors determining the rate and amount absorbed are the drug's ionisation constant and the lipid partition coefficient of the non-ionised moiety.[4]

Surface area of small intestine

Another factor determining drug absorption is the surface area of the small intestine. Normally this is about the size of two tennis courts (doubles size), but its absorptive capacity may be reduced in coeliac disease and some inflammatory bowel conditions. Impaired absorption of digoxin has been found in various malabsorption syndromes, especially coeliac disease. In contrast, most antibiotics are well absorbed in this condition (indeed, absorption may be slightly better than normal), but malabsorption of trimethoprim and clindamycin has been found in jejunal diverticulosis. The pattern of antibiotic absorption is often disturbed in Crohn's disease.[5]

Although local blood supply determines the rate of absorption of drugs given by subcutaneous and intramuscular injection, there is little evidence in man that blood flow to the gut limits absorption, except in patients with cardiogenic shock or gross heart failure.

OTHER FACTORS REDUCING BIOAVAILABILITY

Several other factors may limit the amount of drug reaching the systemic circulation unchanged. Firstly, some drugs, including benzylpenicillin, are destroyed by gastric acid. Secondly, metabolising enzymes are located in the brush border of the small intestine: these include sulphokinases, monoamine oxidase, non-specific esterases, and uridine diphosphate-glucuronyl transferase. The beta-adrenoceptor stimulant drug isoprenaline is extensively metabolised in the intestine, and normally only a small amount reaches the sytemic circulation unchanged. The conjugation of isoprenaline may be reduced by salicylamide, and hence the effects of isoprenaline taken by mouth are increased. Similarly, levodopa is extensively metabolised in the intestine unless given with a decarboxylase inhibitor, and naturally occurring indirect sympathomimetics such as tyramine are normally inactivated in the intestine but may cause hypertensive crises in patients receiving monoamine oxidase inhibitors.

The final obstacle that a drug must traverse before reaching the systemic circulation is the liver. Many lipid-soluble drugs, including beta-adrenoceptor antagonists—such as propranolol and oxprenolol—the analgesics paracetamol and pentazocine, tricyclic antidepressants, and some tranquillisers undergo extensive extraction and biotransformation in this organ. This may lead to major individual differences in the peak levels attained after administration by mouth. This phenomenon is often referred to as a "first-pass effect"; together with variation in the rate of gastric emptying it may lead to major individual differences in response to drugs given by mouth.

DISTRIBUTION

The major factors governing drug distribution are physicochemical, the route of administration, regional blood flow, binding to proteins, and the existence of transport systems; these are, however, interdependent.

Drugs enter the extracellular space by passive diffusion through gaps between the capillary endothelial cells. Thus unless they are too large to diffuse through the pores—in the case of heparin, for example—most drugs will be distributed throughout extracellular fluid. Access to the brain and cerebrospinal fluid (CSF) is, however, limited by the existence of tight junctions between the endothelial cells, which, together with a continuous turnover of CSF and active carrier-mediated outward transport (for instance, penicillin), constitute the blood-brain barrier.[6] Drugs that are extensively un-ionised at physiological pH are freely diffusible across lipoprotein cell membranes and can enter the brain, CSF, and cells throughout the body. Their apparent volume of distribution may therefore be several times that of body water. Lipid-soluble basic drugs, including lignocaine, propranolol, and the tricyclic antidepressants, are widely distributed and concentrate in the tissues, especially brain, liver, and lung. This pattern of distribution may have important consequences in terms of both efficacy and side effects.

Drug distribution is also influenced by the route of administration. Drugs injected intravenously are preferentially distributed to organs and tissues with a high regional blood flow—for example, heart, brain, and kidneys. Thus anaesthesia occurs within seconds of a single intravenous injection of thiopentone because the drug rapidly achieves a high concentration in the brain. But its action is short-lived because subsequent redistribution into other tissues occurs and the concentration in the brain falls below the minimum needed to induce sleep. Similarly, the cardiac effects of drugs start within a minute or less of intravenous injection, and reversion of cardiac arrhythmias often occurs during this time. Fatal arrhythmias, however, may occur when potassium salts are given too rapidly by this route.

Many drugs are carried in blood bound to non-specific sites on plasma proteins, usually albumin. Drug bound to protein is in equilibrium with that free in the plasma water, but only the latter exerts a pharmacological effect. The amount of drug bound to protein is determined by the number of binding sites available (which varies for different drugs), their affinity for the drug, and its concentration. Plasma protein binding is important in drug distribution (and elimination) since only the unbound fraction is available for distribution. Thus the higher the binding of sulphonamides to albumin the greater the proportion that remains in the blood and the lower the concentration in CSF.[7] In the case of diazoxide, 96–98% of which is normally bound to plasma proteins, it is possible to saturate the binding sites by rapid intravenous injection of the drug. This allows the drug to be distributed to sites on vascular smooth muscle and enhances its therapeutic effect. The distribution and efficacy of drugs that are heavily bound to plasma proteins may be influenced by disease, including hypoalbuminaemia caused by cirrhosis of the liver[8] or the nephrotic syndrome. In addition, binding may be abnormal in patients who are uraemic.[9]

Some drugs become highly concentrated in the tissues because their chemical structure allows them to be taken up by selective transport systems. For example, the adrenergic neurone blocking drugs bethanidine, debrisoquine, and guanethidine become concentrated in the adrenergic nerve terminal because they are transported by a system known as uptake.[10] In contrast, the concentration of penicillin in CSF is reduced by a carrier-mediated outward transport that can be blocked by the uricosuric probenecid.[11]

ELIMINATION (INCLUDING INACTIVATION)

The action of many drugs ends with their excretion; possible routes of elimination include pulmonary, renal, biliary, and intestinal. Almost all volatile anaesthetics are excreted, largely unchanged, by the lungs. In addition, the anticonvulsant paraldehyde is partially eliminated by this route. Factors that influence the rate of elimination, therefore, include the effective tidal volume, frequency of ventilation, the solubility of the drug, and ventilation-perfusion relationships in the lung.

Drugs may be handled at three sites in the nephron: they may be filtered at the glomerulus or either secreted by the proximal convoluted tubule or passively reabsorbed from the distal convoluted tubule, or both. Glomerular filtration is determined largely by cardiac output, which in turn relates to plasma volume, but may be reduced by renal disease and in old age. Drugs that undergo active tubular secretion include penicillins, cephalosporins, and probenecid. Most lipid-soluble drugs are almost entirely reabsorbed in the distal nephron by passive diffusion; the latter is pH-dependent and alkalinisation promotes the excretion of phenobarbitone and aspirin, whereas acidification increases the clearance of amphetamine.

Biliary excretion is relatively unimportant for most drugs, because in man the threshold for elimination by this route lies at a molecular weight of about 500 (in contrast to rats, in which the threshold occurs at a molecular weight of 325). None the less, a few drugs do undergo biliary elimination in man, but some—for example, digitoxin and practolol—are reabsorbed from the small intestine, a process referred to as enterohepatic recirculation.

Recently several drugs have been shown to undergo direct elimination across the intestine; they include the beta-adrenoceptor antagonist acebutolol, the antibacterial-antiprotozoal drug metronidazole, and the short-acting cardiac glycoside ouabain. The precise mechanism of this form of excretion is unknown. Small amounts of drugs may be excreted in other fluids, such as breast milk, tears, saliva, and sweat. These routes, however, are quantitatively relatively unimportant and are not considered further.

DRUG METABOLISM

Drugs may be metabolised at many sites but the liver is the most important one. Most drugs are biotransformed by a group of enzymes of relatively low specificity that are also responsible for the degradation of endogenous materials such as bilirubin and hormones. These drug-metabolising enzymes, which are associated with the endoplasmic reticulum, are most active in the liver but exist also in the intestine, kidney, lung, and skin. Pathways of drug metabolism in the microsomal system can broadly be categorised into two main types—firstly, pre-conjugation or phase I reactions, which serve to append or reveal suitable chemical groupings such as OH, NH_2, and COOH within the drug; and, secondly, conjugation or phase II reactions, in which groupings revealed by phase I reactions are coupled to endogenous compounds such as glucuronic acid and sulphate. The end products are more water soluble and can be eliminated in bile or urine. Phase II reactions may occur without prior oxidation, reduction, or hydrolysis if suitable groupings already exist.

Most phase I metabolites are generated by a common hydroxylating enzyme system known as cytochrome P450. The activity of the system is in part genetically determined but is also under the influence of environmental factors including substances present in the diet and various medicines. Drugs may affect the activity of the P450 cytochrome system in one of two ways. Firstly, the amount and activity of the enzyme may be increased by drugs that are referred to as inducers of microsomal oxidation. These include barbiturates, glutethimide, dichloralphenazone (the phenazone fraction), haloperidol, alcohol (in some people), and the antifungal agent griseofulvin. When one of these drugs is introduced into the treatment of a patient stabilised on another that is metabolised by hepatic microsomal enzymes, the effect is to increase gradually the rate of inactivation of the latter. Thus to maintain the previous pharmacological and therapeutic effects it may be necessary to increase the dose twofold or threefold (sometimes tenfold). Other drugs may inhibit the action of hepatic microsomal enzymes and include methylphenidate, chloramphenicol, disulfiram, allopurinol, alcohol (some people), and dextropropoxyphene (in Distalgesic).

Generally phase I reactions lead to a diminution of pharmacological activity, but there are important exceptions to this rule. These include the red dye Prontosil and imipramine, which are converted to the active metabolites sulphanilamide and desipramine respectively. Toxic metabolites of phenacetin and paracetamol may also be generated by this system.

Some phase II reactions take place in the cell sap; among the enzymes located therein, *N*-acetyltransferase is responsible for the acetylation of isoniazid, hydrallazine, sulphonamides, and procainamide. The activity of this enzyme is genetically determined (probably in an autosomal recessive manner), and patients are either fast or slow acetylators. The proportion of the two genotypes varies among ethnic groups; some 95% of Eskimos are fast acetylators whereas among Caucasians the proportion is less than half.

Hydrolysis of some drugs takes place in the blood; non-specific esterases exist in plasma, and these are responsible for the hydrolysis of succinylcholine, procaine, and procainamide. The activity of plasma esterase (pseudocholinesterase) is also genetically determined, but the trimodal distribution in activity suggests an autosomal, autonomous inheritance. Both the heterozygotes and homozygotes for normal enzyme activity hydrolyse succinylcholine rapidly, whereas the homozygotes for the atypical enzyme may suffer from prolonged apnoea after the use of this neuromuscular blocking drug.

CONSEQUENCES OF DIFFERENCES IN BIOAVAILABILITY AND RATES OF ELIMINATION

Despite the convenience of taking drugs by mouth individual differences in the amount of drug reaching the systemic circulation and in the rate of elimination of drug from the body may lead to major differences in response to treatment. Thus average doses quoted in textbooks and the *British National Formulary* should be regarded as optimal for only a proportion of patients. Standard doses may be totally inadequate for some patients, because of either reduced bioavailability or rapid elimination, while in others the same dose may be excessive and cause toxicity.

This article is based on chapter 2 of the author's *Topics in Clinical Pharmacology*. (London, Henry Kimpton. To be published.)

REFERENCES

1 Academy of Pharmaceutical Sciences, *Guidelines for Biopharmaceutical Studies in Man*. Washington, American Pharmaceutical Association, 1972.

[2] Groisser, V W, and Farrar, J T, *Journal of Clinical Investigation*, 1960, **39,** 1607.
[3] Benjamin, D, Robinson, D S, and McCormack, J, *Clinical Research*, 1970, **18,** 336.
[4] Hogben, C A M, *et al*, *Journal of Pharmacology and Experimental Therapeutics*, 1959, **125,** 275.
[5] Parsons, R L, *Hospital Update*, 1976, **2,** 221.
[6] Davson, H, *Journal of Physiology*, 1976, **255,** 1.
[7] Garrod, L P, and O'Grady, F W, *Antibiotic and Chemotherapy*, 3rd edn. Edinburgh and London, Churchill Livingstone, 1971.
[8] Branch, R A, James, J, and Read, A E, *British Journal of Clinical Pharmacology*, 1976, **3,** 243.
[9] Reidenberg, M M, *et al*, *New England Journal of Medicine*, 1971, **285,** 264.
[10] Iversen, L L, *Uptake and Storage of Noradrenaline in Sympathetic Nerves*. London, Cambridge University Press, 1967.
[11] Spector, R, and Lorenzo, A V, *Journal of Pharmacology and Experimental Therapeutics*, 1974, **188,** 55.

Gastrointestinal reactions to drugs

ALEX PATON

By the nature of things few drugs can be entirely free from gastrointestinal side effects, and a glance at the lists of adverse reactions prepared by the Committee on Safety of Medicines[1] will show the impossibility of producing a comprehensive account. The task is somewhat simplified by the fact that relatively few drugs are constant offenders (see table), but the occurrence of new or unexpected gastrointestinal symptoms during the course of treatment should always be viewed with suspicion. Symptoms such as nausea, anorexia, dyspepsia, and diarrhoea are so common that they are all too easily attributed to the illness rather than to the drug.

Drugs commonly associated with gastrointestinal symptoms

Benzodiazepines	Hypotensive agents	Corticosteroids
Antidepressants	Beta-blockers	Oestrogens and progestogens
Appetite suppressants	Digitalis	Oral hypoglycaemic agents
Opium derivatives	Diuretics	Antibiotics
Synthetic analgesics	Theophyllin derivatives	Sulphonamides
Aspirin	Bromhexine hydrochloride	Metronidazole
Anti-inflammatory agents	Iron, calcium, and potassium salts	Cytotoxic agents
Anticholinergic drugs		
Anti-Parkinsonism drugs		

Although some side effects are dose-related, most depend on the sensitivity of the host. This may vary from time to time so that the fact that a particular drug may not have caused trouble on a previous occasion does not ensure its safety. As with all side effects the spectrum of gastrointestinal sensitivity ranges from the person who reacts to a single dose of a drug such as paracetamol that is normally well tolerated, to the patient who, for example, never experiences dyspepsia even with large doses of corticosteroids. While, obviously, drugs that are taken by mouth might be expected to cause gastrointestinal side effects, there is no guarantee that the latter will be avoided by using alternative routes of administration.

Pre-existing disease, such as peptic ulceration, ulcerative colitis, and cardiac failure may predispose to side effects, as may intrinsic defects of the gastrointestinal tract such as gastric atrophy, coeliac disease, and changes brought about by aging.

The following selective account is confined to therapeutic substances, but it should not be forgotten that both nicotine and alcohol produce deleterious effects on the gut.

Gastrointestinal reactions to drugs

THE MOUTH

Most people know that iron and tetracycline may discolour the teeth, but it may not be generally realised that other antibiotics have been reported to do so, as has sodium cromoglycate. Similarly, the effect of phenytoin on the gums is familiar to every medical student, but many other drugs—for example, oestrogens—may be associated with gingivitis. Dryness of the mouth, stomatitis, and glossitis are also common, especially with psychotropic drugs, hypotensive agents, beta-blockers, and antibiotics. Ampicillin and co-trimoxazole may cause ulceration, as may phenylbutazone; and metronidazole is particularly apt to produce glossitis.

NAUSEA AND VOMITING

Six pages of the Committee on Safety of Medicines report[1] are devoted to records of nausea and vomiting. The well-known propensity of opiates to cause vomiting is shared by the newer analgesic compounds —notably, dihydrocodeine, pentazocine and dextropropoxyphene—and by anti-inflammatory drugs. Other substances that are particularly prone to produce nausea and vomiting are anti-Parkinsonism drugs including levodopa, oestrogens and progestogens, cytotoxic agents, bromhexine, and potassium chloride. Of the chemotherapeutic agents, ampicillin, tetracycline, erythromycin, co-trimoxazole, nitrofurantoin, nalidixic acid, and metronidazole are particular offenders. Nausea is the earliest symptom of digitalis intoxication.

DYSPEPSIA

Indigestion may go unremarked because it is so common and with a new drug the relation may not be immediately appreciated. A causative connection between aspirin and dyspepsia is now generally accepted; less so the possibility of acute gastrointestinal haemorrhage, as opposed to chronic blood loss. The rare gastrostaxis is probably a genuine hypersensitivity reaction. It does not seem possible to answer the question whether aspirin has anything to do with perforated peptic ulcer. Most doctors believe that aspirin compounds are potentially dangerous in people with pre-existing oesophagitis, varices, or peptic ulcer. It is necessary only to hold an aspirin tablet against the buccal mucosa until it dissolves to show the harmful effect it has even on normal mucosa.

All compounds containing aspirin are potentially harmful, and the newer formulations have not completely overcome the hazard. It is not always appreciated how many proprietary preparations contain aspirin,[2] some promoted for the relief of indigestion. Paracetamol is safer but weaker and not entirely free from causing dyspepsia and gastrointestinal bleeding. The most dangerous of the anti-inflammatory drugs are undoubtedly phenylbutazone and indomethacin, but they are by far the best anti-inflammatory agents. This seems to be a general correlation: ibuprofen, for example, the least potent of the group, is associated with the least side effects. Of the newer drugs, naproxen already has a reputation for causing gastrointestinal haemorrhage and I would expect it to be a powerful pain reliever.

The gastric dangers of corticosteroids are too well known to need detailed description. The giant ulcer on the greater curve of the stomach is the classical lesion, but any syndrome from hyperacidity and oesophageal reflux to duodenal ulceration may be met with. Dyspepsia occurs with all types of corticosteroids; is to some extent dose-related though still dependent on individual sensitivity; is more likely in people with previous ulcer histories (though this is not necessarily a contraindication to its use); and is said to be commoner in patients with rheumatoid arthritis. Formulations of corticosteroids with drugs like aspirin and phenylbutazone are particularly dangerous.

Various measures can be taken to avoid dyspepsia with these and other drugs. Paracetamol is widely used as an alternative to aspirin but needs to be given in larger doses. Dextropropoxyphene and ethoheptazine, popular for the relief of moderate pain, may also be safer but are not entirely free from side effects. The routine use of alkalis when the more powerful anti-inflammatory drugs or corticosteroids are being used has been recommended; some drugs—for example, phenylbutazone—can be obtained with alkali incorporated. Enteric-coated preparations of aspirin, phenylbutazone, and prednisolone are available but are considerably more expensive and may cause trouble in the small bowel where they dissolve; they should be reserved for patients known to be sensitive to the ordinary preparations. Serious confusion has resulted from failure to appreciate that enteric-coated prednisolone tablets are only half the strength of the usual prednisolone. Suppositories of indomethacin are widely used, but even this route does not entirely avoid dyspepsia, and a local proctitis may follow long-continued use. Parenteral administration of corticosteroids or corticotrophin does not prevent gastric side effects, adding weight to the view that their action is not solely a local one. Tablets of all these drugs should, of course, be taken with food.

ALTERATION IN BOWELS HABIT

We tend to forget that many commonly used drugs may affect the bowels. Magnesium trisilicate is a powerful laxative, while aluminium salts are constipating. Hypotensive drugs often constipate, though guanethidine and methyldopa may cause diarrhoea. Antibiotics of all sorts are apt to loosen the bowels, and serious forms of enterocolitis (pseudomembranous colitis) often with bacterial superinfection have followed the use of newer drugs such as clindamycin and lincomycin, though they were not unknown with previous broad-spectrum antibiotics. Less threatening forms of diarrhoea probably result from alteration of the bowel flora, and fungal infection may supervene. Purgative abuse, with characteristic appearances on barium enema examination and sometimes an Addisonian-like picture, should always be considered as a cause of unexplained diarrhoea.

Anti-inflammatory agents, especially the fenamic acid derivatives, appetite suppressants, and sex hormones may all cause diarrhoea, as may digitalis and diuretics. Digitalis can also produce a syndrome resembling mesenteric occlusion, with pain and bloody diarrhoea, especially in the elderly, while thiazide diuretics have been reported to induce an allergic vasculitis affecting the small bowel. Salts of iron, calcium, and potassium have an irritant effect on the bowel. Enteric-coated potassium chloride had a predilection for causing ulceration of the small bowel, usually manifest as obstruction, but occasionally as perforation or haemorrhage. This effect is said to have been abolished by the introduction of slow-release tablets, but these may still cause similar lesions—for example, in the oesophagus—as a result of hold-up.

Steatorrhoea has been observed after the use of drugs, some predictable, like neomycin, cholestyramine, and cytotoxic agents, others less so, such as phenindione, para-aminosalicylic acid, and mefenamic acid. Some drugs interfere with the absorption of essential factors such as vitamin B_{12} and folid acid.[3]

Constipation may be a problem with opiates, psychotropic drugs, anticholinergic agents, hypotensives, and iron. Ileus has been reported with some of these, especially antidepressants; and perforation is a particularly dangerous complication of corticosteroid treatment, since symptoms are often masked by the drug.

ENVOI

A great deal of discomfort and much needless investigation might be avoided if we were always to consider the possibility of drugs being the cause of a patient's gastrointestinal symptoms.

REFERENCES

1 Committee on Safety of Medicines, *Register of Adverse Reactions*, vol III. London, Department of Health and Social Security, 1974.

2 Banks, C N, and Baron, J H, *Lancet*, 1964, **1**, 1165.

3 Clark, F, *Adverse Drug Reaction Bulletin*, 1976, **57**, 196.

View from general practice

J G R HOWIE

In general practice alimentary diseases form the smallest proportion of diseases of the major systems that can be classified in traditional hospital terms, but the largest proportion (nearly one-third) of those handled on a symptomatic basis. The recent national study of morbidity seen in general practice[1] recorded only some 4% of all episodes of illness as caused by classifiable disorders of the system, with a further 4% of episodes grouped under the category of unclassified symptoms relating to the digestive tract. When the wide variations among doctors in their preferences for disease as against symptom labelling is also considered, it can be seen that the difficulty in deciding whether to discuss diseases or symptoms becomes a major one.

Before considering treatment it is reasonable to look at the figures already quoted in terms which reflect the day-to-day work of family doctors. One patient in 12 will present a disorder of the alimentary system, and this will represent three or four consultations during the average day. Nearly half will be acute diarrhoea or vomiting. Dyspeptic illness is next commonest, patients in this category being seen at the rate of perhaps two a week. Depending on policies of investigation, half will have proved ulcers, half suspected ulcers. Most of these patients will not be consulting for the first time with such symptoms. During the course of a year an average of some 20 patients will present with each of the diagnoses aphthous ulcer, dental abscess or caries, hernia, fissure, haemorrhoids, and constipation, although many more will have laxatives prescribed without regular consultation. Except in epidemics, jaundice is a rare condition. From the total of undifferentiated illnesses that include abdominal pain as a symptom (most alimentary complaints are in this category) possible appendicitis is probably diagnosed less often than once a month (and confirmed as correct in terms of needing surgery in half these cases); acute gall bladder disease is about equally prevalent. New diagnoses such as perforated ulcer, haematemesis, ulcerative colitis, obstruction, carcinoma of stomach, carcinoma of colon, and carcinoma of rectum are made no more than once or twice each during an average year.

The general practitioner thus carries into his thinking about treatment of alimentary disease three groups of disorders; the first is of common disorders, difficult to define in precise aetiological or diagnostic terms but usually benign and often self-limiting; the second contains comparatively uncommon conditions that are often materially inconveniencing, fairly easily defined, and usually treatable; and the third is composed of rare but serious conditions that need early recognition for saving life.

TREATMENT

It is all too easy to equate "treatment" in general practice with prescribing drugs. While many useful therapeutic agents are available, drugs have a comparatively limited contribution to make to managing patients with alimentary illness. Some general approaches to management may be considered briefly before discussing the treatment of some of the commoner presentations of alimentary disease.

Advice and education

Certainly, the commonest presenting symptom—diarrhoea—may usually be managed expectantly. Numerous consultations result from patients eating too much too soon after diarrhoeal illness, and many others reflect patient experience of receiving unnecessary medication on previous occasions. Simple advice on starvation and intake of fluid will treat most acute episodes adequately—especially in adults. In addition, it forms the basis of encouraging the self-treatment—which most doctors adopt themselves—of future episodes. At the other extreme, non-specific constipation is more healthily treated by increasing dietary fibre than by laxatives, and many patients still need to be convinced that regularity and frequency are not synonyms.

Dyspepsia is as appropriately managed by reducing consumption of chips, alcohol, and cigarettes as increasing intake of alkalis; and the recurrence of haemorrhoids and fissures may be prevented by avoiding constipation. Doctors often complain of the high attendance rates for minor illness of certain patients. How often do they ask if they themselves are in greater or lesser part responsible through having failed to provide necessary health education and by having confirmed the appropriateness of consulting behaviour by prescribing non-essential drugs?

Observation

Eventually diagnosis, and therefore treatment, depend on identifying recognised patterns of natural history of illness. The more points on the progress of a symptom-sign complex that can be charted, the easier it becomes to define the disorder; the less the interference by drug-taking, the greater the probability that the observations made will reflect the underlying illness and its progress. Thus vomiting that continues is more apt to be caused by, for example, jaundice than is vomiting that stops after four hours; new dyspepsia that persists is more likely to indicate malignancy than is recurrent dyspepsia that remits; alterations of bowel habit may come to be capable of interpretation or—sometimes significantly—may fail to conform to known disease patterns and the acute abdomen, the greatest cause of anxiety to most general practitioners, may develop into clearly recognisable obstetric, surgical, or medical conditions. Active observation[2] is indeed a positive form of treatment.

Investigation

When it is realised that at least half the disorders of this system are dealt with symptomatically, the importance of knowing when investigation should be part of the management plan becomes axiomatic. Attempts to convert all symptomatic diagnoses to disease diagnoses on the basis of investigation would quickly overwhelm bacteriological, biochemical, radiological, and outpatient resources with relatively small return to the health of the general community or individual patient. The new and apparently increasing range of endoscopic investigations available, together with the possibilities of new and specific treatments becoming available for various conditions not particularly amenable to treatment (such as peptic ulcer), make definition of appropriate rules of investigation hazardous. Is the barium meal examination about to become outdated? Is it correct that general practitioners in some centres should have been discouraged or refused access to barium enema investigation because sigmoidoscopy was thought an essential concomitant investigation? If so why do regional differences apply? What is the place of liver biopsy?

Can we guarantee that when our patients are investigated the number of uncomfortable, undignified, and sometimes frightening procedures in the package is kept to a minimum—and that each is explained fully? At the other extreme, the teaching that management of diarrhoea requires stool culture so patently demonstrates lack of realism that specific investigation of at-risk groups (food handlers, babies, those in institutions, for example) is now often inappropriately neglected, and relevant clinical and epidemiological information is lost.

Referral

The previous section will have hinted at my growing feeling that the investigation of resistant alimentary problems should normally be carried out (where geographically realistic) by a carefully briefed specialist. Serious alimentary disease is seen too rarely for general practitioners to develop real skill in the use of diagnostic aids, and the consequences of under-diagnosis are important. As well as issues covered in the previous section, referral for rectal bleeding (to be differentiated from anal bleeding) is regarded by many as mandatory; but general practitioners would appreciate a specialist consensus on whether proctoscopy in the surgery is sufficient investigation, or whether hospital sigmoidoscopy should be added routinely for definable groups of such patients.

View from general practice

The acute abdomen—the commonest cause of referral to hospital for *any* general practice condition—must be under specialist supervision when appreciable diagnostic uncertainty is present; but the specialist must be briefed adequately on (and respond constructively to) the many non-physical features that may have material bearing on the long-term handling of the individual patient.

Prescription

Few articles make more interesting contemporary reading than that by Dunlop and his colleagues[3] on general practitioner prescribing of over 20 years ago. Then cholagogues, bitters, and antacids were the second commonest group of drugs prescribed. In Patterson's more recent review of general practice prescribing,[4] hypnotics and psychotropic drugs, antibiotics, drugs acting on the respiratory system, analgesics and antirheumatics, and topical preparations were all more often prescribed than gastrointestinal medications—although the range of different preparations used was exceeded only by topical preparations and the combined grouping of hypnotic and psychotropic drugs. The *Monthly Index of Medical Specialties* (*MIMS*) lists 38 antacids, 53 gastrointestinal sedatives, 38 laxatives, purgatives, or lubricants, 22 preparations acting locally on the rectum, and 36 antidiarrhoeals (two-thirds still containing an antibiotic or sulphonamide). The *British National Formulary* (*BNF*) lists a total of 36 formulations to cover all these headings. (An additional 18 preparations for nausea and vomiting are listed in *MIMS* and nine in the *BNF*.)

The range of preparations indicates the widespread use of symptomatic medication and the absence in some cases of specific treatment and in other cases of clear market leaders. As in so many areas of general practice prescribing, personal choice of doctor or patient tends to dominate therapeutic principle.

SOME PERSONAL POLICIES

Symptomatic and self-limiting conditions

The three principal illnesses in the symptomatic and self-limiting conditions group are diarrhoea (with or without vomiting), dyspepsia, and constipation. My view is that, in all three, patient education is the principal therapeutic agent and accordingly explanation and advice dominate my approach to management. Starvation and fluid replacement are the centre-pieces in managing diarrhoea; few people continue to be sick for more than a few hours and really troublesome diarrhoea and colic normally settle quickly. Few preparations probably make much difference to ability to continue at work but when this is a consideration kaolin and morphine may be tried. Antibiotics are *not* part of treatment. Dyspepsia normally responds to diet including bland foods and milk and excluding fats, cigarettes, and spirits. Stress must be identified, discussed, and when possible reduced.

Many patients have their favourite antacid and that I would normally prescribe on request; my own choice is usually magnesium trisilicate compound mixture (BPC) or the popular proprietary Aludrox (aluminium hydroxide gel). At present the places of carbenoxolone, the new liquorice and bismuth preparations, and the radically new histamine receptor antagonist, cimetidine, are being evaluated in carefully designed and controlled studies. I would prefer to support these projects by referring appropriate patients to specialists organising the projects (after explanation to the patients) rather than initiate treatment, the results of which can be assessed only subjectively outside proper research protocols. Resistant dyspepsia requires referral; close observation may, however, be needed to allow resistant dyspepsia to be recognised; changing drugs may confuse rather than clarify this important issue.

In its chronic form constipation is often much helped by heeding the message of the bran promoters. Advice to introduce bran to the diet, together with education as to the real range of normal bowel habit, is probably the most constructive approach to treatment. Personally, I recommend laxatives only in the presence of other lesions that may be aggravated by constipation (disc lesions and anal fissure, for example). Like most other doctors, however, I prescribe them much more often than I recommend them.

Readily defined and inconveniencing disorders

Disorders in the readily defined and inconveniencing disorders category can be comparatively easily visualised and are found principally at the extremes of the tract. Mouth ulcers are uncomfortable and for some patients a recurring problem. Choline salicylate (Bonjela) is an inexpensive and popular remedy for this. Dental infections are most appropriately treated with penicillin by mouth; advice to seek dental treatment is part of proper care, and telephone communication with a dental colleague promotes much useful goodwill.

At the other end of the tract, pruritus ani—remarkably common and most uncomfortable—responds readily to almost any soothing local application, but steroids appear particularly helpful. In treating anal fissure one of several preparations containing steroid, local anaesthetic, and topical antibiotic or antiseptic will provide quick relief. My own particular choice is one of the more expensive of these preparations; I have no good reason for persisting in using it: the name just always comes to mind first, often the true reason for a particular therapeutic choice. Haemorrhoids may be treated similarly, suppositories perhaps being used in conjunction with ointments. The value of ice-packs and raising the foot of the bed, especially when a thombrosis of an external pile is threatening, is also of value. Referral for surgical opinion must always be considered but assessment of individual cases rather than blanket generalisations should be the rule.

Uncommon and life-threatening conditions

Little comment about uncommon and life-threatening conditions beyond that in earlier sections of this review is needed. The unexplained acute abdomen, the possible malignancy, the persisting diarrhoea, and the unexplained jaundice or weight loss are only further confused by dabbling in medication. Consultation (in its true sense) with specialists should be an early policy. Until the need for this becomes evident, careful serial observation is, of course, the best indicator of the range of possible disorders.

NON-PHYSICAL ILLNESS

No view from general practice would be complete without referring to the recurring dilemma of the general practitioner—namely, the need to balance physical disease and its appropriate management against psychological or social illness and its appropriate management. The presentation of non-physical disease in terms of physical disease is a well-known phenomenon of general practice, although doctors vary widely in their interpretation of (and even ability to recognise) different patterns of illness behaviour. Obesity (usually) and weight loss (often) may reflect depression or anxiety, and altered bowel habit and abdominal pain may also be due to psychological rather than physical factors.

Here again my belief—increasingly firmly held—is that prescribing drugs and initiating investigations should not be seen as the automatic first approach to these problems. It is often relatively easy to identify patients for whom planned observation together with a sympathetic but probing interviewing technique should be given a real chance to get behind the headlines. It may be that only when fundamental emotional problems have been identified can effective treatment be planned.

CONCLUSION

Disease of the alimentary system is important but diffuse. Classification and diagnosis are difficult; thus discussion of management must be more subjective and personal than it might ideally be. Emphasis has been on management strategies rather than on specific disorders and remedies. The review of symptoms, diseases, and treatments is not all-embracing (hiatus hernia, malabsorption, diverticulitis, and other conditions have not been mentioned), but I have tried to develop three main themes.

Firstly, much disease of the alimentary system is best thought of in symptomatic terms and treated by advice and better patient education. The general practitioner needs, however, close (and mutually informed) relations with relevant specialists so that new advances in diagnostic thinking and treatment can be brought to the benefit of the right patients in the most efficient way possible.

Secondly, several readily definable and inconveniencing conditions occur often enough to require the family doctor to be familiar with appropriate policies for their treatment. What the individual doctor chooses will represent a personal choice from a wide (unnecessarily wide, I believe) range of available preparations, some apparently more therapeutically supportable than others.

Thirdly, some diseases with sinister potential are seen too infrequently to allow the general practitioner any reasonable chance of gaining necessary expertise in their investigation or acute management. Consultation, referral, and observation are the appropriate management tactics for these.

REFERENCES

1 Office of Population Censuses and Surveys, *Morbidity Statistics from General Practice. Studies on Medical and Population Subjects No 26.* London, HMSO, 1974.
2 Jones, P F, *British Medical Journal*, 1976, **3**, 551.
3 Dunlop, D M, Henderson, T L, and Inch, R S, *British Medical Journal*, 1952, **1**, 292.
4 Patterson, J S, *Journal of the Royal College of General Practitioners*, 1972, **22**, 191.

Nausea and vomiting

DENIS GIBBS

Complex processes underlie the symptoms of nausea and vomiting. Presumably these mechanisms evolved to the organism's advantage. Boyle observed three centuries ago that "'tis profitable for man that his stomach should nauseate and reject things that have a loathsome taste or smell."[1] Nevertheless, though the stomach may sometimes empty itself of certain noxious substances when this is required, nausea and vomiting often seem to serve no discernibly useful function. Seasickness, the commonest form of motion sickness, may be considered as an example. Its importance is emphasised by the fact that the word nausea is derived from the Greek for a ship. Analysis of the sufferer's symptoms and signs conveys a picture of complex autonomic changes. Pallor, coldness, sweating, salivation, nausea, and anorexia precede vomiting. In addition, there may be drowsiness, headache, and lassitude. It is impossible to conceive any advantage for the sufferer once he has embarked from the security of terra firma; and the imagination is stretched to impute a teleologically protective role to seasickness as a means of curbing exploratory and adventurous instincts.

To treat the symptoms of nausea and vomiting rationally, a comprehensive diagnosis should have been established; the susceptibility and circumstances of the individual assessed; and possible hazards and disadvantages of symptomatic approaches considered. There are many conditions in which symptomatic treatment is not appropriate—for instance, nausea and vomiting are common accompaniments of abdominal disorders needing surgical treatment; or vomiting, sometimes without nausea, may be a feature of raised intracranial pressure. Similarly, when the symptoms are derived from metabolic or drug-induced disturbances, treatment of the underlying abnormality or withdrawal of a drug, rather than symptomatic measures, is needed.

Vomiting, particularly when forceful and accompanied by strain and retching, may itself have harmful consequences. The eponymous Mallory-Weiss and Boerhaave syndromes represent the most dramatic results of violent vomiting. Longitudinally placed laceration in the lower oesophagus, with resulting haemorrhage, occurs in the Mallory-Weiss syndrome, typically in someone who has had an alcoholic binge. But indulgence in alcohol is not a prerequisite for such lesions, which sometimes occur after strenuous vomiting for other reasons; patients with small sliding hiatus hernias are susceptible. Boerhaave's syndrome is an extremely rare catastrophe in which violent vomiting causes rupture of the oesophagus.

There are more prosaic but much more common consequences of vomiting. After abdominal surgery undue vomiting may interrupt recovery by delaying or preventing wound healing; or after ocular surgery sudden movement and changes in pressure may lead to vitreous loss. More generally, prolonged vomiting from whatever cause inevitably results in fluid and electrolyte loss, and among various consequences such depletion is then likely to perpetuate the symptoms of nausea and vomiting.

CENTRES AND PATHWAYS CONCERNED WITH VOMITING

Drugs that suppress or modify the symptoms of nausea and vomiting act at various sites; these may be discussed in terms of neurological pathways and centres, so far as they are understood. Firstly, psychological stimuli to nausea and vomiting may be initiated by sights, smells, or associations peculiar to the person, and these are subserved by cortical pathways. Secondly, reflex stimuli operate from abdominal organs via both vagal and sympathetic afferent nerves. Thirdly, impulses originating from the vestibular organs are the primary cause of motion sickness. Fourthly, there are many compounds such as apomorphine, morphine, ergot derivatives, digitalis glycosides, nitrogen mustards, and probably numerous metabolites, that produce their effects humorally, acting directly on areas in the medulla.

The vomiting centre is in the reticular core of the medulla; its function is now thought to be one of co-ordinating various components in the act of vomiting. Many other centres exist close to the vomiting centre. They include a spasmodic respiratory centre, inspiratory and expiratory centres, vasomotor centre, salivatory nuclei, and bulbofacilitatory and inhibitory systems. The process of vomiting may need action by all these centres under the co-ordinating influence of the vomiting centre. On the medullary surface next to the vomiting centre is a second area known as the chemoreceptor trigger zone that responds to various compounds and transmits impulses to the vomiting centre. Many stimuli to vomit are transmitted directly from visceral organs to the vomiting centre and are independent of the chemoreceptor trigger zone. Vagal fibres are usually considered to be more important than sympathetic pathways; they, for instance, conduct impulses that start vomiting in patients with abdominal distension.

The actions of various emetics have been studied and illustrate the variety and complexity of possible effects. As an example, copper sulphate given by mouth in small quantities provokes impulses from receptors in the stomach that are then conveyed to the vomiting centre via both sympathetic and vagal fibres. In larger amounts copper sulphate when absorbed imposes a central action by directly stimulating the chemoreceptor zone. In other instances long-held assumptions have been challenged—for example, staphylococcal enterotoxin was thought to induce vomiting mainly by central actions, whereas its effect is now known to be primarily peripheral, on the gut.

INDIVIDUAL SUSCEPTIBILITY

Wide differences exist between individuals' susceptibility to conditions that cause nausea and vomiting. Most people are seasick in rough conditions, but they acquire tolerance within a few days and then lose their symptoms completely. A few fortunate people are never affected and, at the other extreme, some remain highly susceptible. Another variation in vulnerability is that after surgical operations. "Postanaesthetic vomiting" occurs more commonly in women than men, is more likely after long operations, and decreases in frequency with advancing age.

The threshold of response of the chemoreceptor trigger zone is thought to be influenced by blood levels of certain hormones. Raised levels of oestrogen are considered to play a part in sickness of pregnancy, and in those who develop nausea when they first take oral contraceptives. Synthetic oestrogen given, for instance, in the treatment of prostatic carcinoma may cause similar symptoms. Greater understanding of the basis for differences in susceptibility to vomiting between the sexes and in different groups of people may lead to more effective therapeutic approaches. At present, however, the important practical implication of such differences lies in the special attention needed by those who are particularly vulnerable. In such people there is justification for prophylactic treatment and, if necessary, they may have to avoid anything particularly likely to induce sickness.

ANTIEMETIC DRUGS

Four categories of drugs are valuable in the symptomatic alleviation or prevention of nausea and vomiting: anticholinergic drugs, antihistamines, derivatives of phenothiazine, and an orthopramide drug, metoclopramide. The actions of these drugs are seldom confined to one site; but atropine-like substances and certain antihistaminic substances act mainly on the vomiting centre, whereas the phenothiazines primarily influence the chemoreceptor trigger zone.

Hyoscine—Anticholinergic drugs have long been known for their antiemetic effects particularly in preventing or relieving motion sickness. In trials during the second world war hyoscine hydrobromide proved the most effective. Hyoscine has atropine-like actions, but it is also a central nervous depressant. In benefiting motion sickness the anticholinergic action by which it blocks afferent impulses at the vomiting centre is important, but its cortical effects and also probably some peripheral influence on the labyrinth also contribute to its effectiveness. In therapeutic doses (0·6–0·9 mg) side effects are likely to include some drowsiness, slight headache, dryness of the mouth, and inability to read small print. The susceptible traveller usually considers these effects a small price to pay for the prevention of motion sickness. But caution is required in the elderly, in whom transient mental confusion may occur. A child under 5 years old may need 0·15 mg before travelling, though young children are, in fact, often less susceptible than their parents to the effects of motion. Children from 5–15 may need adult doses, but half-doses are usually sufficient.

Antihistamines—The discovery that an antihistamine drug had antiemetic effects provides an interesting example of serendipity. Dimenhydrinate (Dramamine) was sent for clinical trial to the allergy clinic of the Johns Hopkins Hospital. During treatment with this drug a patient with urticaria noticed that she no longer suffered from car sickness. Dimenhydrinate was then given to USA troops crossing the Atlantic in the *General Ballou*, a rather top-heavy converted freight ship. Though it was found to be valuable in preventing seasickness, initial impressions were over-enthusiastic, and later trials failed to show any striking superiority over other remedies—particularly hyoscine.

Dimenhydrinate was thus established as the first antihistaminic drug shown to have antiemetic properties. Such properties are not common to all antihistamine preparations; the activity is specific, mainly by direct sedation of the vomiting centre, and is independent of the other actions of the drugs concerned. There is no direct correlation between the central effects of particular antihistaminic preparations and their potency as peripheral histamine antagonists. The antihistamine drugs that help motion sickness are also of some value in treating the nausea and vomiting caused by labyrinthine disturbances such as labyrinthitis and fenestration operations. The vomiting produced by apomorphine is scarcely affected, as the chemoreceptor trigger zone is not suppressed by these drugs. Examples of antihistamine drugs with antiemetic activity include: dimenhydrinate (Dramamine), cyclizine hydrochloride (Valoid), promethazine hydrochloride (Phenergan), and meclozine hydrochloride (Ancolan), the latter two being longer-acting than the former. The antihistamine drugs often induce drowsiness and unsteadiness that are enhanced by alcohol.

Phenothiazines—Those phenothiazine derivatives that possess antiemetic activity act primarily in blocking the chemoreceptor trigger zone. They exert general sedative effects as well, but there is little impact on the vomiting centre. This accounts for the fact that though impulses pass through the chemoreceptor trigger zone en route from the vestibular organs to the vomiting centre, phenothiazine derivatives have not proved particularly useful in treating motion sickness.

Nausea and vomiting

Chlorpromazine in relatively low and non-sedative doses was found to prevent vomiting that would otherwise be induced by agents acting on the chemoreceptor trigger zone. This prompt and specific action is exerted either by competition for the receptor site or by a directly depressive effect on this area in the medulla. This potent and selective action has many useful clinical applications in conditions such as uraemia, carcinomatosis, radiation sickness, and in helping to counteract the nauseating effects of many drugs.

There has been no convincing demonstration of a greater antiemetic efficacy of one phenothiazine congener over another, but chlorpromazine is regarded as less suitable than some newer compounds because of the greater risk of jaundice. Advantages of the newer compounds are partly offset by a greater likelihood of inducing extrapyramidal effects. Examples of piperazine side-chain phenothiazines that have potent antiemetic activity include perphenazine (Fentazin), prochlorperazine (Stemetil), and thiethylperazine maleate (Torecan). The extrapyramidal side effects shown by oculogyric crises and muscle rigidity may render these drugs unsuitable for repeated administration in some patients.

Metoclopramide—Metoclopramide is a drug with unique actions in the upper gastrointestinal tract. It was synthesised in France from a derivative of procaine and then applied clinically in conditions associated with dysfunction in the gastroduodenojejunal area. Studies in many parts of the world subsequently confirmed that it possessed powerful antiemetic properties with an order of activity similar to the phenothiazines. In man it causes a rise in pressure at the lower oesophageal sphincter, increases both the frequency and amplitude of gastric contractions, and speeds the rate of transit through the small bowel. In patients with duodenal ulcers it accelerates gastric emptying, both of liquids and of isotope mixed with solid food. These actions render it pharmacologically distinct from other compounds in therapeutic use.

Other recent clinical studies on particular groups of patients who are apt to vomit owing to gastric retention are relevant. For instance, metoclopramide has been reported to improve delayed gastric emptying in diabetics. It also benefits gastric retention after gastric surgery. Observations on patients who have had antrectomies are relevant. One suggestion had been that a major action of metoclopramide in accelerating gastric emptying was by increasing the closeness of synchronisation between antral and duodenal contractions. Its efficacy in patients in whom the antrum had been removed indicates that it cannot solely act in that way. In fact, the mechanisms of its action remain poorly understood and debate continues even whether its effect is mediated mainly through nerves or directly on muscle. Studies in animals have also indicated some action on the chemoreceptor trigger zone, but undoubtedly the clinically important actions in man are on the motility of the upper gastrointestinal tract. Its limited central action is illustrated by its relative ineffectiveness in motion sickness. Metoclopramide does not cause frequent side effects, but lassitude and drowsiness sometimes occur when the drug is given in therapeutic doses, and occasionally extrapyramidal reactions are seen. In the adult such reactions are usually a consequence of taking too much of the drug.

THERAPEUTIC APPROACHES

Motion sickness

In both the prevention and treatment of motion sickness, when exposure is likely to last only a few hours, hyoscine hydrobromide is the most satisfactory drug (tab hyoscine *BP* 0·3 mg). Two tablets (0·6 mg) should be taken an hour before exposure to the motion and thereafter 0·3 mg may be taken at six-hourly intervals. Doubling the dose is more effective but other consequences, notably dryness of the mouth and drowsiness, are more evident. In prolonged exposure an antihistaminic drug, such as diphenhydramine 50 mg three times a day, or meclozine 50 mg once or twice daily, is preferred, with an expected 50–60% success rate. Such drugs may be continued for several days while tolerance to the motion is acquired. In some people who do not have responsibilities while travelling the sedative effects of cyclizine are desirable, in a dose up to 50 mg three times a day. Alcohol should be avoided while taking either hyoscine or an antihistamine preparation.

In the poor sailor both physical and psychological factors are relevant. Many people find their own remedies: they learn to avoid overindulgence in food and alcohol, shun stuffy cabins and nauseating smells, and avoid the company of those already afflicted. By remaining amidships they are less likely to be affected, and some rely on fixing their gaze on the horizon as a means of maintaining a stable posture.

Nausea and vomiting of pregnancy

An important physical basis for pregnancy sickness may exist in alterations in levels of hormones, but the use of neither hormonal nor antihormonal agents is at present feasible. In current concepts of management special emphasis is placed on the application of conventional general measures. These include encouragement and psychological support and the correction of nutritional and electrolyte imbalance. The doctor must ensure that the patient is taking frequent small meals rich in carbohydrate, and that her fluid intake is adequate. Ideally no drugs should be given during the first trimester. There are, however, occasions when a pregnant woman is so nauseated and anorexic that an antihistamine preparation or phenothiazine derivative is considered justifiable. Features such as weight loss, dehydration, or the restriction of normal activities provide a mandate for using such drugs.

Nausea and vomiting

No well-controlled trial has shown one agent to be more effective than another.

When drug treatment is deemed essential it is usual to start with an antihistamine such as meclozine, promethazine, or trimethobenzamide, whereas those with severe nausea and vomiting and those who do not respond are given one of the newer piperazine side-chain phenothiazines. Chlorpromazine is considered less suitable than the newer compounds because of the slightly greater risk of inducing jaundice; but if there is associated epilepsy or suspected eclampsia the newer phenothiazine congeners are best avoided because of their tendency to produce extrapyramidal effects.

In patients with severe vomiting of pregenancy physical and psychological influences are difficult to separate. In addition, in any one person there is a small possibility that a disorder unconnected with the pregnancy may be contributing to the illness. The occasional presence of a disturbance such as raised intracranial pressure, peptic ulceration, hepatitis, drug reactions, and cholecystitis is easily overlooked.

Postoperative nausea and vomiting

The decrease in incidence of postanaesthetic nausea and vomiting has been attributed to the use of new anaesthetics, greater attention to efficient ventilation and hydration, and a greater awareness of the part played by opiate drugs used in premedication. In ill patients undergoing major surgery there may be dangerous side effects from some antiemetic drugs, especially hypotension. Routine prophylactic treatment with antiemetics is not indicated. In addition, opiates given postoperatively for pain, rather than included in the premedication regimen, cause less nausea and vomiting.

When antiemetic treatment is needed postoperatively three choices in drug treatment are available: (*a*) the antihistaminic drugs such as cyclizine and promethazine are only moderately effective but have the advantage of relative non-toxicity; (*b*) the piperazine side-chain phenothiazines, such as perphanazine and prochlorperazine are more potent but cause more side effects, with drowsiness, hypotension, and extrapyramidal symptoms liable to complicate the postoperative condition; and (*c*) metoclopramide is helpful in some patients and in the adult carries little risk of side effects. Metoclopramide is particularly valuable in reducing the risk of vomiting preoperatively or during induction of anaesthesia—for instance, for surgery in the casualty department or for a patient in labour.

Toxic and drug-induced nausea and vomiting

Nausea and vomiting in patients undergoing treatment for neoplastic diseases may be related in part to the underlying illness, but often the treatment is solely responsible. Virtually all patients given nitrogen mustard preparations have nausea, and about half of these will be subject to severe vomiting, which begins one to three hours after treatment. Cyclizine and promethazine provide partial control of the nausea and vomiting that follow treatment with cytotoxic drugs, but many patients are more effectively relieved by the more potent phenothiazine derivatives. Prophylactic administration given just before the cytotoxic agent is usually desirable.

Miscellaneous causes

Acute vomiting and diarrhoea caused by various pathogens, many of which are assumed to be viral, constitute one of the commonest diseases in the community. Antiemetic drugs are not of value in the symptomatic control of gastroenteritis. Cyclizine, however, has a place in controlling the persistent nausea which is often such an unpleasant accompaniment of hepatitis.

Several ototoxic agents including streptomycin affect the vestibular apparatus giving rise to vertigo, nausea, and vomiting; inner ear disease including Menière's disease, neuronitis, postural vertigo, and eighth-nerve tumours may have similar effects. Destructive middle ear disease and surgical procedures on the middle ear may also damage the inner ear and result in a symptom complex in which vertigo is dominant and which is accompanied by nausea. Dizziness and nausea may be helped by antihistamine drugs such as dimenhydrinate, cyclizine, or meclozine.

Patients suffering from Menière's disease causing frequent attacks may benefit from betahistine. This histamine analogue was developed because the parenteral use of histamine reduced the symptoms of vertigo and tinnitus in Menière's disease. Betahistine probably exerts its effect by reducing endolymphatic pressure. Antihistamines should not be used concurrently. Symptoms of nausea and headaches, as well as exacerbation of peptic ulceration, have occasionally been reported in patients receiving betahistine.

New surgical procedures are being devised to combat inner ear disease and may have to be considered in patients suffering from severe vertigo, nausea, and vomiting of inner ear origin. In some such patients the repeated administration of antiemetic drugs, including new phenothiazine derivatives, is justified even when there is the risk of causing extrapyramidal side effects.

CONCLUSIONS

Ryle observed that "symptoms are a part of morbid physiology; they express disturbances of function. As a rule, therefore, they precede the development of signs which are but the outward morbid anatomy of the living." He chose nausea as one of three symptoms to illustrate his thesis. Since the publication of his *Natural History of Disease*, the opportunities and expectations of symptomatic treatment of nausea and vomiting have greatly increased. There should be a concomitant increase in diagnostic precision if the doctor is to avoid inappropriate application of symptomatic drugs. In addition, it is evident that the sites and modes of action of antiemetic drugs are incompletely understood and that their side effects are often unpleasant and occasionally dangerous.

REFERENCES

[1] Boyle, R, *Vulgarly Received Notions of Nature*. London, Taylor, 1686.
[2] Ryle, J A, *The Natural History of Disease*, 2nd edn. London, Oxford University Press, 1948.

Pain

LAURENCE M BLENDIS

Pain in the alimentary system may be divided into oesophageal pain and abdominal pain.

OESOPHAGEAL PAIN

Heartburn

Heartburn is a retrosternal burning sensation, often worse on lying down or bending over and commonly associated with a sour or acid taste in the mouth. The symptom is caused by gastric acid reflux into the oesophagus through an incompetent cardiac sphincter. The diagnosis may be confirmed by a barium meal examination provided the cardiac sphincter mechanism is challenged by various manoeuvres. If the history is suggestive of reflux it is important not to be deterred by a normal barium meal result since the examination may have been inadequate and, in addition, incompetence of the cardiac sphincter may be intermittent.

Treatment consists of important common-sense measures such as removal of tight abdominal garments and appreciable weight reduction when necessary, together with small regular meals and, for nocturnal heartburn, raising the head of the bed. In addition, regular antacid treatment is usually needed, such as 10–15 ml or tablets of alternating magnesium trisilicate and aluminium hydroxide every two hours. More resistant cases may need metaclopramide, 10 mg three to four times a day by mouth. This drug probably increases cardiac sphincter pressure and gastric emptying and is virtually free of side effects. Medication may often be gradually reduced over two to three months. If the symptoms persist or need maximum medication, surgery may be considered, particularly in the presence of a hiatal hernia.

Dysphagia

Dysphagia (pain or difficulty, or both, on swallowing) most commonly occurs in patients with peptic oesophagitis secondary to acid reflux. It is diagnosed for certain by oesophagoscopy with or without the aid of biopsies, but it is important to exclude a peptic stricture in these patients since this indicates a further stage of the disease.

The symptoms may respond to measures described above, but these patients are more likely to need surgery, particularly if a stricture is present and even if it responds initially to dilatation. Dysphagia, however, especially in the absence of preceding reflux, should always be carefully investigated to exclude malignancy.

Pain

Oesophageal spasm

Classically, oesophageal spasm is a severe retrosternal pain that may last for up to a minute or so but may leave a residual soreness. It may be difficult, however, to differentiate it from cardiac pain, and often it is diagnosed by exclusion after performing chest radiographs and electrocardiograms. Medical treatment is extremely difficult. Smooth muscle relaxants such as amyl nitrite, octyl nitrite, glyceryl trinitrate, and longer-acting nitrites have been tried without much success.

ABDOMINAL PAIN

Anterior abdominal wall

In many patients complaining of abdominal pain it is important to differentiate pain originating in the structures of the abdominal wall from that within the peritoneal cavity. In the former, the patient may give a history of physical strain or the pain may be related to activity or standing and is relieved by resting. A tender area may be located that can be shown to be in the abdominal wall when the patient tenses the abdominal muscles. The possibility of a small ventral hernia must be considered.

Rest and treatment with an analgesic such as paracetamol is often sufficient. In contrast, anterior abdominal wall pain may be associated with a lax abdominal wall and is often considerably helped by an anterior support garment.

Upper abdominal pain

Upper abdominal pain may originate from the stomach, the transverse colon, or the gall bladder. The clinical differentiation of peptic ulcer from non-organic pain may be difficult.

Peptic ulcer—Classically, peptic ulcer pain is periodic, often waking the patient at night, and is associated with hunger that is partially relieved by meals. The diagnosis is confirmed by a barium meal examination or endoscopy. If both examination results are negative but the symptoms are highly suggestive of peptic ulcer and persist repeat examinations must be performed. Symptoms are often helped by eating something every two hours throughout the day and avoiding large meals, late suppers, and spicy foods or concentrated alcohol. This, together with regular antacids every two hours throughout the day, with a double dose of 20 ml last thing at night form the basis of medical treatment. Anticholinergics such as poldine or propantheline tablets may be added if symptoms are not controlled. To achieve the desired effect of considerably reducing gastric acid secretion, however, they must be given up to maximally tolerated doses, that is poldine 4 mg up to six times a day. This is assessed by side effects such as dryness of the mouth and blurring of vision and this treatment is contraindicated in patients with prostatism. Since these drugs tend to cause constipation, they are best used with magnesium trisilicate or hydroxide as the antacid.

In chronic gastric ulceration, carbenoxolone sodium, at a maximum dose of 100 mg three times daily, promotes healing of the ulcer. No such evidence exists for chronic duodenal ulceration. Carbenoxolone has major aldosterone-like properties and may thus cause major side effects of salt and water retention, with oedema and kaliuresis with hypokalaemia. It is therefore contraindicated in patients with congestive cardiac failure and hypertension, and patients on this drug must be regularly weighed every other day and examined weekly for side effects. Treatment usually lasts about six weeks.

Non-organic pain—In contrast, constant abdominal pain or discomfort that shows no constant relationship with meals and does not wake the patient at night is likely to be of the so-called non-organic type. This pain is often associated with persistent nausea, abdominal distention, and belching suggesting aerophagy as a cause, and these latter symptoms may be reproduced by gastric distention with air during gastroscopy. On examination, however, the patient may have the same degree of upper abdominal tenderness as a peptic ulcer patient. It is often diagnosed by excluding organic disease, and a follow-up study of a large group of well-investigated patients with 'barium-negative dyspepsia' found that less than 2% subsequently developed an organic lesion.

Gall bladder—The only symptom that is definitely associated with gall bladder disease is that of biliary colic. Acute attacks of colicky pain in the right upper quadrant with or without associated dark urine or clinical jaundice are caused by a gall stone in the cystic or bile duct. The waves of pain are severe, inducing sweating, and powerful analgesia such as pentazocine or pethidine are often needed for relief.

In a recent series of patients undergoing cholecystectomy, however, the site of pain (which disappeared postoperatively) varied from the right iliac fossa to the left upper quadrant. Other symptoms such as fat intolerance, nausea, and flatulence are no more frequent than in control populations. At present, the medical treatment of gall stones by dissolution with chenodeoxycholic acid should be carried out only at designated centres.

Left-sided abdominal pain

Colonic pain may occur anywhere over the distribution of the colon, but the commonest sites are the left iliac fossa and left side of the abdomen, central upper abdomen, and then right and left upper quadrants. Colonic pain is caused by disorders of motility. In young adults this is most commonly caused by the irritable bowel syndrome, in which the main symptoms are pain and early morning diarrhoea, often with a normal bowel action later in the day.

The pain is constant with fluctuations during the day, rarely waking the patient at night, and persisting for years. It is aggravated by many factors such as eating, smoking, stress, or menstruation. Unfortunately, it is usually diagnosed by exclusion necessitating sigmoidoscopy, a barium enema, often additional *x*-ray examinations, an examination under anaesthesia or dilatation and curettage, and not infrequently negative laparotomy. This results in an undue delay of the correct management, which is first and foremost a sympathetic doctor who understands the nature of the pain, is prepared to explain it to the patient, and to continue the management over a long period. In addition, a high fibre diet often helps. This may vary from added bran one to three times a day and wholemeal bread to a diet rich in vegetables and salads. Antispasmodics such as mebeverine 100–200 mg four times a day for at least three to six months, may help. Finally, transquillisers or antidepressants should be used only when clearly indicated.

Diverticular disease—The pain associated with diverticular disease is nearly always localised to the left iliac fossa and is associated with constipation. Both these symptoms respond remarkably to a high fibre diet. In contrast, the pain of acute diverticulitis, which is associated with fever and leucocytosis, needs anticholinergics, antibiotics, and a low residue diet until the attack has subsided.

Central abdominal pain

Chronic pancreatitis—Pain associated with chronic pancreatitis is perhaps the most severe form of chronic abdominal pain. Classically it radiates through to the back and may be relieved by sitting forward. It is diagnosed principally by radiology, in which calcification in the region of the pancreas is virtually diagnostic. The results of barium *x*-ray examinations are disappointing but the newer technique of endoscopic retrograde pancreatography after cannulation of the ampulla of Vater under direct vision is a considerable advance. Unfortunately, after diagnosis, medical treatment has little to offer apart from increasing the strength of the analgesic.

Abdominal angina—Another type of pain in the central abdomen is associated with large as opposed to small meals and sometimes with exercise. Called abdominal angina, it is associated with ischaemia either of the coeliac axis or superior mesenteric artery, and is an important diagnosis to consider. The one doubtful physical sign is that of a loud arterial bruit over the affected artery. Arteriography can show a narrowing of the vessel, and trinitrin sublingually may relieve the pain. If medical measures fail surgery must be considered, but results will depend on the type of lesion, the size of vessel affected, and many other factors.

Acute abdomen—It is beyond the scope of this article to deal with the differential diagnosis of pain associated with the acute abdomen. In the more chronic forms of abdominal pain, however, even when a specific remedy is available it is important to treat the whole patient in terms of his personality and background and always to consider diet, which invariably plays an important part in managing abdominal pain.

FURTHER READING

Harvey, R F, Pomare, E W, and Heaton, K W, *Lancet*, 1973, **1**, 1278.
Hill, O W, and Blendis, L, *Gut*, 1967, **8**, 221.
Palmer, W L, *et al*, *Postgraduate Medical Journal*, 1974, **50**, 416.
Waller, S L, and Misiewicz, J J, *Lancet*, 1969, **2**, 753.

Haematemesis and melaena

P B COTTON, R C G RUSSELL

Acute gastrointestinal haemorrhage remains a common cause of emergency hospital admission, with a mortality close to 10% despite recent improvements in resuscitation, anaesthesia, and surgery.[1] In Britain, most patients bleed from peptic ulcers or from erosions of the stomach or oesophagus.[2] The range of potential sources is large, however, and includes varices, tumours, mucosal tears, vascular malformations, and foreign bodies. The outlook for an individual patient depends upon the source of the bleeding, age, and the presence of co-existing disease.[3]

We see few patients who bleed so copiously that on admission they need immediate surgery to prevent exsanguination. Most stop spontaneously, if only temporarily. This brief respite allows resuscitation, assessment, and the formation of a management plan, bearing in mind an overall chance of immediate rebleeding of around 20%. There is a delicate balance to be drawn between conservatism and aggression, in both diagnosis and treatment.

ASSESSMENT

In Britain, most bleeding patients are initially admitted to medical wards. This is logical, because of the high incidence of concomitant disease and its important effect on prognosis, but the admitting physician must be aware of the natural history of haemorrhage and of the dangers of a leisurely approach. Management by a combined medicosurgical gastrointestinal team is a rarely achieved ideal. In most hospitals patients will be handled by the general admitting medical and surgical teams, whose specialist interest may lie elsewhere. The advantage of a multidisciplinary approach to severely ill patients has been highlighted and enhanced by the development of intensive treatment units, and it is logical to admit all severe bleeders to them for two or three days. The analogy of myocardial infarction and coronary care units is quite close. There is a critical period of about 72 hours when close observation and quick co-operative decisions are essential. Many patients who bleed are young and should have a normal expectation of life after the episode, which cannot be said for the young patient with coronary disease.

When faced with a patient believed to have bled, there are four basic questions: (1) How much has the patient bled? (2) Where has the blood come from? (3) What else is wrong with the patient, and how will he stand up to resuscitation, investigation, rebleeding, or surgery? and (4) What should be done?

Blood loss

While patients often overestimate the amount of blood lost, the doctors' common error is to underestimate it, because of the body's compensatory mechanisms. There is no routine place for blood volume measurement, but there is often an urgent need to replace volume as guided by careful sequential observation. Arbitrary definitions of a major bleed are always open to criticism, but anyone who needs volume replacement immediately on admission to hospital, or who has serious co-existent disease, is certainly at high risk.

At the other end of the scale some patients who claim to have vomited blood are mistaken or malingering, and not all black material is sanguine. Blood from the teeth or nasopharynx may be swallowed overnight and vomited in the morning, particularly by children. Consideration of these possibilities may sometimes prevent unnecessary investigation and even hospital admission.

Sources of bleeding

More than 90% of patients presenting with haematemesis or melaena, or both, have a lesion proximal to the papilla of Vater. Nevertheless, some presenting with malaena alone have a more distal lesion, sometimes even in the colon. The clinical history and physical examination, though important, are poor guides to the precise origin. Since peptic ulcers are the most common source, inquiry about previous dyspepsia or ulcer disease should always be made. The answer, however, may be misleading. Twenty-five per cent of patients with chronic dyspepsia are not bleeding from ulcers, and 30% of those with bleeding ulcers deny previous dyspepsia.[2] Recent salicylate ingestion without previous dyspepsia is often taken to suggest acute gastric erosions, particularly in the presence of a negative barium meal result, but this assumption is quite wrong, Salicylate ingestion is so common that many patients with this history are equally likely to be bleeding from a chronic ulcer.

It is fortunate, because treatment is so unsatisfactory, that oesophageal varices are a rare cause of bleeding (about 3%). Here again the history may be misleading. It has been shown repeatedly that patients with known cirrhosis or known oesophageal varices may be bleeding from other sources (ulcers and erosions). Knowledge of a congenital or acquired coagulation problem is relevant to management but does not define the site of bleeding; the same is true for patients known to have telangiectasia or other arteriovenous malformations.

Two particular clinical histories are helpful in suggesting the source of bleeding. A small red haematemesis after repeated and forceful vomiting strongly suggests a Mallory-Weiss tear of the oesophagogastric junction, although such a history may be present in only half the patients with this condition. Bleeding from severe oesophagitis is seen quite often in elderly patients who are confined to bed because of intercurrent illness or recent surgery. In retrospect most admit to a history of heartburn. Until bleeding oesophagitis is diagnosed the condition may even be aggravated by raising the foot of the bed in an attempt to maintain central perfusion—a procedure to be deprecated in any event. Most patients stop bleeding quickly once the diagnosis is determined and the correct posture maintained.

Endoscopy

Thus clinical history and examination rarely provide a precise diagnosis of the bleeding source. Until recently diagnostic attempts relied upon the barium meal examination, supplemented in a few centres by gastroscopy. Many patients came to laparotomy without a precise diagnosis, and some indeed to necropsy. This unsatisfactory state of affairs is currently changing with the spread of fibreoptic oesophago-gastroduodenoscopy.[4] In experienced hands, upper gastrointestinal endoscopy is highly accurate in diagnosing both large and small lesions. In all hospitals with a good endoscopy service this has become the procedure of first choice in investigating bleeding patients, and most radiologists would agree that the barium meal examination is a second best.[5] Urgent endoscopy is not universally available, however, and expert barium radiology is certainly much better than inexperienced endoscopy.

The correct timing for diagnostic investigation is a matter of judgment and availability. Emergency endoscopy within a few hours of admission is difficult to arrange, but delay beyond 48 hours is illogical, since many patients will already have rebled. In the average case we have compromised by examining patients within 12 to 18 hours. If major haemorrhage has occurred and early surgical intervention is being considered endoscopy is performed sooner, though here the likelihood of blood obscuring the endoscopic view is quite high and cannot always be overcome by gastric lavage. We have often found it appropriate to examine such patients in the anaesthetic room of the operating theatre, under a general anaesthetic, with the surgeon in attendance. This allows a good examination and comprehensive gastric lavage if necessary. At the very least, it enables the endoscopist to exclude a bleeding oesophageal lesion.

If endoscopy fails to define a bleeding lesion and haemorrhage persists urgent arteriography by an expert may be helpful.[6] Vascular malformations are particularly well demonstrated by this technique, which also has potential therapeutic applications (intra-arterial infusion of adrenalin, of vasopressin, or embolism with clots) in certain contexts. A prior barium meal examination will render angiography impossible.

Most endoscopic series provide an overall positive diagnosis in

80–90%. Gastric and duodenal ulcers together provide around 50%, and acute mucosal lesions another 15–20%. One of the lessons of widespread fibreoptic endoscopy is that duodenal ulceration is rather less important as a bleeding source, and oesophagitis and Mallory-Weiss lesions rather more, than was previously thought.[4] In all endoscopic series there is a substantial group (10–25%) of patients who are found to have more than one potential bleeding lesion. A patient with a duodenal ulcer may in fact bleed from acute erosions or a mucosal tear. Herein lies a major advantage of endoscopy over barium studies, since it is usually possible to tell at endoscopy where the blood is coming from. In a few patients the result of the examination is entirely negative and no blood is seen, which suggests that the source is distal to the ampulla of Vater and that further diagnostic steps should be considered such as sigmoidoscopy, arteriography, barium enema, or colonoscopy.

General state of health

The clinical history and physical examination in a bleeding patient should lead to a comprehensive knowledge of the patient's health, both past and present. Concomitant renal or cardiopulmonary disease will greatly affect decisions about patient management and the eventual prognosis. A few patients present with bleeding as a terminal event of an incurable malignant disease.

The assessment of any patient with a major bleed should be as rigorous as that of a patient admitted to an intensive care unit with a myocardial infarction. Baseline haematology and chemistry are important, and a clotting screen will often be necessary. Chest radiography and an electrocardiogram shortly after admission may identify previously unsuspected risk factors and provide invaluable baselines, as may blood gas analyses.

MANAGEMENT PLAN

On the basis of the foregoing comprehensive assessment, it should be possible to formulate a plan of action, including the likelihood of surgical intervention. For a minor bleeding episode from an acute mucosal lesion patients may only need inpatient observation for a few days, along with oral alkalis. There is no indication of any dietary restriction. Management of a major bleeding episode is more complex.

MANAGEMENT OF A MAJOR BLEED[7]

Patients need careful observation, and the use of an intensive treatment area has already been recommended. Replacement by blood, or occasionally blood substitutes, remains of prime importance, but the speed of replacement and need for supportive medication such as digoxin or diuretics must be determined for each patient. Particularly in the elderly patient with associated disease, blind replacement of blood is no longer acceptable. Careful monitoring of the central venous pressure, hourly urine output, and changes in the electrocardiogram may all be necessary if full advantage is to be taken of the opportunities provided by an early diagnosis. Electrolyte abnormalities, hypoproteinaemia, coagulation deficiencies, vitamin deficiencies, and anoxia may all need correction. The objective of the resuscitation period should be to prepare the patient for a further bleed or surgery.

Unnecessary delay and unnecessary surgery are both dangerous. An early accurate diagnosis should define a path between these chasms. The "blind gastrectomy" should now have passed into the history of surgery. Nearly all surface mucosal lesions (oesophagitis, Mallory-Weiss syndrome, acute erosions) stop bleeding spontaneously. Oesophageal varices often rebleed but surgery carries a formidable risk. The surgeons' main contribution lies with patients bleeding from peptic ulcers or neoplasms.

Peptic ulcer—If a patient is bleeding from a peptic ulcer and has a long past history of ulceration, surgery is usually offered as soon as the resuscitation phase is complete. In the same patient with the same ulcer, but no previous history, there is a tendency to await a second bleed. While this appears logical, several series have shown that patients with no previous history are at greater risk,[1 3] presumably because of this tendency to delay surgery. It is often stated that rebleeding is more likely in the older age group. This may simply reflect the higher incidence of gastric to duodenal ulceration. It is also true, however, that the mortality of surgery increases with advancing age. Thus judgment in the individual case is a question of balancing risks. It is certainly true that the operative mortality rises with delay, and most authorities recommend early operation in the elderly bleeder once chronic ulceration is established. A bleeding anastomotic ulcer usually needs early surgery.

For bleeding gastric ulceration most surgeons favour a Billroth I gastrectomy with excision of the ulcer. The correct procedure for a bleeding duodenal ulcer remains debatable. Best results are obtained by the surgeon performing the operation with which he is most familiar. Reports suggest that a Polya gastrectomy is more effective in preventing rebleeding but has a higher mortality than vagotomy and drainage. The trend is towards vagotomy with under-running of the bleeding vessel through the pyloroplasty. Whether the vagotomy is truncal or selective is a matter of individual experience. Proximal gastric vagotomy is not to be advocated in an emergency. Nevertheless, advocates of this technique may employ it on an early elective basis after conservative management of the bleeding episode if the latter has not been severe, and the main indication for surgery is the chronicity of ulceration.

Gastric neoplasm—In the rare patient who bleeds acutely from a gastric neoplasm, surgical delay will serve no purpose once the initial assessment has been carried out, excepting that the patient's chance of short- and long-term survival after major resection will depend upon the availability of an appropriate surgeon.

Acute mucosal lesions—Despite the overall good prognosis for patients bleeding from acute mucosal lesions a few continue to bleed. Until recently surgery provided the only possible treatment. Most surgeons would perform a Billroth I gastrectomy with or without vagotomy, with a commitment to total gastrectomy if bleeding persisted. Radical surgery after days of intensive medical management and repeated blood transfusions carries a formidable mortality. It is for these patients that the new acid-suppressing drugs such as cimetidine (see below) will have important application.

Hiatus hernia itself is not a cause of bleeding. Occasionally gastric ulcers occur at the level of the diaphragmatic hiatus, but in most cases bleeding results from acute reflux oesophagitis. This virtually always stops when alkalis are given and the patient is propped up. Surgical intervention may sometimes be appropriate after recovery from the bleeding episode.

Oesophageal varices—The patient with bleeding oesophageal varices poses a formidable problem[8] with which few surgeons are experienced. The acute episode is usually managed medically with replacement of blood and clotting factors, intravenous or arterial infusions of vasopressin, and a Sengstaken-Blakemore tube, along with the usual measures to alleviate or prevent hepatic insufficiency. This type of regimen usually provides temporary control. Failure needs a more aggressive approach, either directly on the oesophagus or through a shunt procedure. Sclerosis of varices can be performed through an oesophagoscope or through transhepatic catheterisation of the coronary vein. The choice of a shunt procedure remains controversial, and will in any event depend upon a radiological assessment of the portal system. There has been recent enthusiasm for mesocaval shunting using a Dacron graft. The complexity of management of these patients is such that their best chance of survival lies in units with special interest and competence in the condition; if patients are to be referred to such a centre it should be done early, while the patient is still relatively fit.

Rare causes—There are many rare causes of haematemesis and melaena. The investigation and management of these patients is often prolonged and punctuated by negative investigations, even laparotomy. Careful angiography is sometimes diagnostic. When laparotomy is to be performed on a patient with recurrent undiagnosed bleeding, on-table transintestinal endoscopy should be considered; with the abdomen open, it is easy to thread a fibreoptic endoscope through the entire small intestine and obtain excellent views on withdrawal. The Zollinger-Ellison syndrome should not be forgotten as a cause of rebleeding, particularly after surgery. An urgent serum gastrin estimation may be diagnostic.

POSTOPERATIVE MANAGEMENT

Careful postoperative care in an intensive treatment area is vital. In the elderly group of patients after major surgery, the commonest problems are those of pulmonary embolism, cerebrovascular and coronary episodes, as well as respiratory problems. The maintenance of normal perfusion and oxygenation is often of critical importance, and planned intermittent positive pressure ventilation may be appropriate immediately after operation. The incidence of pulmonary embolism may be reduced by low-dose subcutaneous heparin starting immediately before operation. Accurate fluid replacement is essential, and early physiotherapy and avoidance of a nasogastric tube can do much to prevent chest complications. Parenteral nutrition may be necessary.

NEW THERAPEUTIC DEVELOPMENTS

The management of certain patients with acute upper gastrointestinal bleeding may well be altered by developments that are under evaluation. Gastric acid secretion may be virtually abolished by the H^2 blocking agent cimetidine. This treatment can certainly help in the management of patients with bleeding mucosal erosions[9] and in the Zollinger-Ellison syndrome. Its precise application in other bleeding patients is under trial.

The second development concerns the local treatment of bleeding lesions through fibreoptic endoscopes.[10] Injection of sclerosants into varices has already been mentioned. Diathermy coagulation can be applied to erosions, angiomas, and small ulcers. A laser beam has been used for the same purpose. An endoscope has been produced with which it is possible to apply clips to bleeding vessels. These applications are experimental and are unlikely to find widespread application. Small lesions usually stop bleeding spontaneously, and large ones usually require surgery.

ASSESSMENT OF RESULTS

It seems reasonably to hope that careful assessment, accurate diagnosis, urgent resuscitation, careful observation, and skilful selected surgery will result in benefit to individual patients. To prove any such benefit, or to assess the contribution of any single factor, is much more difficult.[11] It is often stated that the overall mortality of haematemesis and melaena has changed little over many years. Different series, however, contain a different spectrum of lesions; the age of patients and their load of concomitant disease may well be changing.[12] A static overall mortality may obscure improvements in one area, and indeed adverse trends in another. Now that it is possible to diagnose precisely in most cases, we can assess the efficacy of our treatment within each diagnostic category and institute trials of different therapeutic protocols. Only in this way will progress or failure become apparent.

REFERENCES

1 Schiller, K F R, Truelove, S C, and Gwyn Williams, G, *British Medical Journal*, 1970, **1**, 7.
2 Cotton, P B, *et al*, *British Medical Journal*, 1973, **2**, 505.
3 Johnston, S J, *et al*, *British Medical Journal*, 1973, **3**, 655.
4 Cotton, P B, in *Topics in Gastroenterology: 3*, ed S C Truelove and M J Goodman. London, Blackwell Scientific, 1975.
5 Stevenson, G W, Cox, R R, and Roberts, C J C, *British Medical Journal*, 1976, **2**, 723.
6 Irving, J D, and Northfield, T C, *British Medical Journal*, 1976, **1**, 929.
7 *British Medical Journal*, 1974, **1**, 403.
8 *Lancet*, 1976, **1**, 846.
9 MacDonald, A S, Steele, B J, and Bottomley, M G, *Lancet*, 1976, **1**, 68.
10 Katon, R M, *Gastroenterology*, 1976, **70**, 272.
11 Logan, R F A, and Finlayson, N D C, *Lancet*, 1976, **1**, 1173.
12 Allan, R, and Dykes, P, *Quarterly Journal of Medicine*, 1976, **45**, 533.

Dysphagia

MICHAEL ATKINSON

Dysphagia must always be taken seriously, not only because it usually indicates serious disease but because in itself it often has dire consequences. As a symptom, at the best it is an embarrassment that detracts from the pleasures of the table and may disrupt social life for fear of eating in public; at the worst it threatens existence by causing starvation or respiratory complications. Although life may be maintained for varying periods by feeding either intravenously or through a gastrostomy or jejunostomy, in the long term these methods are poor substitutes for being able to swallow one's food. The rational management of dysphagia must be based on a proper understanding of the nature of the derangement that is present and of the possible consequences of being unable to swallow.

MECHANISM OF DYSPHAGIA

Swallowing is a complex reflex, the initial stages of which are under voluntary control; hence it is absent in the unconscious patient. The reflex is initiated by compressing the bolus between the tongue and the hard palate, thus pushing solids into the pharynx and squirting liquid down into the lower oesophagus. Difficulty in initiating swallowing may result from paralysis of the tongue muscles, palatal damage, and painful lesions in the mouth and throat including those after traumas or surgery in this area.

Weakness of the pharyngeal constrictor muscles retards the rate of passage of the bolus through the throat, and ineffective closing off of the larynx and nasopharynx allows some to enter the respiratory tree causing coughing and choking or regurgitation of fluids through the nose. The constrictor muscles receive their motor supply from the nucleus ambiguus, damage to which from brain stem ischaemia, poliomyelitis, motor neurone disease, or syringobulbia causes pharyngeal dysphagia.

Upper oesophagitis, which may or may not be associated with web formation, occurs because iron deficiency causes atrophic changes in the mucosa, which make it vulnerable to minor trauma from food. As with peptic oesophagitis in the lower oesophagus, mucosal irritation leads to spasm of the underlying oesophageal muscle that obstructs the passage of the bolus.

Loss of oesophageal peristalsis occurs with advancing years and in systemic sclerosis, but dysphagia from this cause is usually mild provided the patient swallows when sitting or standing, when gravity helps transit. Under these conditions liquids pass readily down the oesophagus and when peristalsis is weak or absent dysphagia usually occurs only with solid foods. Radiological examination shows that swallowed contrast medium remains in the oesophagus for minutes or even hours when the patient is examined in the recumbent or 15° head down position. Effective peristalsis may also be disrupted by neuromuscular incoordination, as in oesophageal spasm or achalasia. Here there is no organic obstruction, but the failure of the lower oesophageal sphincter or of the oesophagus to relax when the bolus arrives coupled with the absence of co-ordinated propulsion higher in the gullet causes dysphagia. Fortunately the upper oesophageal sphincter (cricopharyngeus) is unaffected in these disorders and protects against regurgitation of retained oesophageal contents into the pharynx and respiratory tree.

Mechanically obstructive lesions such as neoplasm or peptic stricture occurring anywhere between the throat and the upper part of the stomach cause dysphagia. The degree of hold-up depends not only on the diameter of the residual lumen but also on the force and co-ordination of peristalsis higher in the oesophagus. In disorders such as systemic sclerosis and in old age peristalsis may be weak or lacking and so a peptic stricture or neoplasm may cause severe dysphagia for solids before luminal narrowing is gross. The storage capacity of the oesophagus above an obstructing lesion in its lower part is usually sufficient to prevent choking on the first swallow and a sense of hold-up deters the patient from taking more food.

CONSEQUENCES OF DYSPHAGIA

Starvation

The body needs a constant source of energy to support its metabolic processes and to maintain the life of its cells. Food intake provides this energy source and in its absence body fat reserves are used to provide metabolic fuel in the form of free fatty acids and ketones. Glucose for metabolism, however, is mainly provided by the breakdown of body protein, particularly that of muscle, and administered glucose has a considerable protein sparing effect. Surgical operations and radiotherapy increase body protein breakdown and thus accentuate the effects of starvation. On the other hand, correction of under-nutrition enables the patient to tolerate more easily these procedures that may be necessary to deal with the cause of his dysphagia. Starvation impairs wound healing, reduces resistance to infections, and depresses immune responsiveness, all of which increase morbidity and mortality.

If immediate relief of dysphagia is impossible measures to correct under-nutrition should be instituted promptly. If a nasogastric tube can be passed, feeding by this means is preferable to intravenous feeding. Homogenised ward food may be used, but more accurate control of the patient's intake of calories, nitrogen, and electrolytes may be obtained by using a specially made feed consisting of a glucose polymer (Caloreen) 600 g, a beef serum hydrolysate (Albumaid) 60 g, 1 egg yolk to provide essential fatty acids, plus vitamins and minerals made up to 1500 ml of water and given over 24 hours. Appropriate adjustment to the composition of the feed must be made in the presence of hypercatabolism or electrolyte imbalance. Intravenous feeding combining an amino-acid solution, a fat emulsion, and fructose, glucose, sorbiton, or ethanol to provide calories is needed only in patients in whom nasogastric feeding is impracticable because of difficulty in passing the tube or associated disturbance of gastrointestinal function. If the problem persists such patients in the longer term need a feeding gastrostomy or jejunostomy, but fortunately these procedures are now rarely used.

Respiratory complications

Disorder of the pharyngeal phase of swallowing often causes food and liquids to enter the respiratory tract; when the hold-up is in the middle or lower oesophagus regurgitation of oesophageal content is particularly likely to occur at night causing staining of the pillow or during the induction of anaesthesia. In the elderly patient after mild regurgitation has continued for some time the larynx becomes less sensitive to foreign material, and at radiological examination barium contrast medium may enter the larynx and trachea without causing undue distress.

Acute massive aspiration of oesophageal contents is often fatal, although lacking gastric juice and bile the aspirated material is less irritant than vomit. The risk of aspiration during anaesthesia may be reduced by allowing only clear fluids by mouth for several days beforehand, by aspirating the oesophageal contents while the patient is still conscious, and by the rapid insertion of a cuffed endotracheal tube after induction.

Chronic aspiration is much commoner and leads to aspiration pneumonitis, bronchiectasis, and pulmonary fibrosis. Chronic cough, wheezing, and increased breathlessness on exertion are the presenting symptoms and on occasion may overshadow those of the underlying lesion. Aspiration pneumonitis appears in the chest *x*-ray picture as a patchy shadowing usually in the mid-zones, and it is more frequent in the right lung. Mycobacteria derived from food may appear in the sputum and lead to a mistaken diagnosis of tuberculosis. Lung abscess is a serious but fortunately now uncommon complication. The best preventative for aspiration pneumonitis is effective treatment of the underlying cause of dysphagia, but the risk may be diminished by avoiding meals for three hours before retiring and by sleeping with the head of the bed raised on 10-cm blocks.

Carcinoma of the oesophagus

Carcinoma of the oesophagus occurs seven times more often in patients with longstanding achalasia than in the general population. Probably stasis and consequent oesophagitis are the major factors accounting for this association. There is an increased incidence of postcricoid and upper oesophageal carcinoma in sideropenic dysphagia.

MANAGEMENT OF DYSPHAGIA

Unconsciousness

Injudicious attempts at feeding the comatose patient by mouth may lead to respiratory complications, and those who remain unconscious for long periods, as for example after brain damage, should be fed by a nasogastric route.

Oropharyngeal disease

Dryness of the mouth or oropharyngeal infections make swallowing difficult. Lack of saliva in Sjögren's syndrome (keratoconjunctivitis sicca) may cause mild difficulty in swallowing and can usually be helped by taking plenty of liquids with meals and by sucking acid drops. Stomatitis caused by monilial infections, herpes simplex, Stevens-Johnson syndrome, and throat infections may cause severe dysphagia sufficient to result in fluid imbalance. The treatment here is that of the specific infection. Extensive aphthous ulceration can make eating painful, and the topical application of a local anaesthetic (benzocaine lozenges *BPC*) or triamcinolone in oral paste (Adcortyl in Orabase) before meals is of value. Dysphagia due to pharyngeal pouch or post-cricoid carcinoma is usually relieved by appropriate treatment of its cause, but if the resulting nutritional disturbance is great preliminary nasogastric feeding is worth while.

Neuromuscular disorders of the pharynx

Although nasogastric feeding is sometimes needed in the early stages of the lateral medullary syndrome, sufficient recovery usually ensues for this to be discontinued after a week or two. Dysphagia in chronic bulbar palsy and dystrophia myotonica is progressive and difficult to manage; aspiration into the respiratory tract is common in the later stages and may necessitate tracheostomy. Dysphagia in myasthenia gravis usually responds dramatically to neostigmine, which should be given before meals.

Sideropenic dysphagia

Repletion of the body's iron stores alleviates sideropenic dysphagia, but added anxiety is often an aggravating factor and reassurance and tranquillising drugs are then helpful in improving swallowing.

Dysphagia

Achalasia

There is no way in which normal function can be restored to the achalasic oesophagus, and treatment aims at disrupting the circular muscle fibres of the lower oesophageal sphincter by either cardiomyotomy or bag dilatation. Bouginage has no place in managing this disorder because its effects are transient. Effective treatment of achalasia not only restores swallowing to near normal and so improves nutrition but by abolishing oesophageal stasis removes the risk of respiratory complications. Whether effective treatment diminishes the likelihood of carcinoma developing is uncertain, and this complication may arise after successful cardiomyotomy.

Cardiomyotomy is the treatment of choice for achalasia, and most surgeons prefer a transthoracic approach and an incision through the muscle coat to expose the mucosa carried upwards for 8 to 10 cm from just distal to the cardia. A good result is obtained in 80 to 90% of patients, and complications are few, although in a minority gastro-oesophageal reflux is a troublesome sequel. The operation is advisable even in patients with mild or moderate dysphagia and minimal weight loss, because of the likelihood of the condition progressing and the risks of respiratory complications.

Bag dilatation gives a less permanent cure and is best reserved for those patients who are unfit for operation on grounds of age or other disability. If the disease has progressed to the stage of causing advance starvation then bag dilatation may be useful as a temporary measure to restore satisfactory swallowing and so enable nutrition to be improved before undertaking cardiomyotomy. A mechanical dilator (Starck), or hydrostatic (Plummer) or pneumatic (Rieder Moeller) bags, may be used, and they are best introduced along a guidewire threaded through the cardia under direct fibre-endoscopic vision that checks the final position of the bag radiologically. Distention to a pressure of 250 mm Hg for two minutes is adequate to rupture many of the circular muscle fibres of the lower oesophageal sphincter. Good results may be expected in 60% of patients, but the procedure often has to be repeated several times.

Although these procedures open up the cardia, they do not restore normal oesophageal peristalsis. Transit through the oesophagus is largely dependent on gravity, and swallowing in recumbency causes oesophageal stasis.

Peptic oesophageal stricture

Treatment of peptic oesophageal stricture has two objectives: the first to dilate the stricture and so relieve dysphagia, and the second to control gastro-oesophageal reflux and so prevent the stricture reforming.

Dilatation is best done using either solid bougies pushed down the lumen of the rigid oesophagoscope or olive dilators mounted on a flexible carrier and passed over a guiding string or wire that has been inserted through the stricture. Peptic strictures can conveniently be dilated using fibreoptic endoscopy and the Eder-Peustow olive dilators. Under direct vision a guidewire is inserted through the stricture into the stomach. The wire may be difficult to pass in patients with much distortion and angulation of the strictured area, and also it may be held up at diaphragmatic level in those with hiatal hernias. Radiological screening using a mobile image intensifier is helpful in these cases.

When the wire is in position the scope is removed, and olive dilators of increasing size mounted on a flexible carrier are passed over it and through the stricture up to a No 45 French (14·5 mm diameter) olive. The wire is then removed and the scope reinserted, when it will usually pass through the dilated stricture allowing full visualisation of its whole extent and allowing adequate biopsy specimens to be taken. This is important because neoplastic strictures may closely resemble peptic strictures in their radiological and endoscopic appearances. A careful endoscopic search of the stomach, pylorus, and first and second parts of the duodenum is made to detect associated peptic ulcer or fibrotic narrowing that may be aggravating gastro-oesophageal reflux. The examination can be done under local anaesthesia using intravenous diazepam supplemented by pethidine if the patient develops pain. General anaesthesia using a cuffed endotracheal tube is preferable in children, uncooperative patients, and those with tight strictures or considerable food residues in the oesophagus. When this method is used perforation and mediastinitis occur in under 2% of dilatations.

The frequency with which oesophageal dilatation has to be repeated varies greatly from patient to patient and is largely determined by the efficacy of treatment to control reflux. Since most peptic strictures occur in the elderly, the reflux is usually treated medically and this comprises sleeping with the head of the bed raised on 10-cm blocks, regular antacids combined with dimethicone (Asilone Gel) and metoclopramide to improve cesophageal clearance together with getting the patient to lose weight and stop smoking. Control of gastric secretion with the H_2 antagonist cimetidine offers hope of reducing oesophagitis and restricturing. Careful mastication is important in the presence of oesophageal narrowing, and some elderly edentulous patients prefer to homogenise their food.

Surgical measures to control reflux should be considered in younger patients with symptoms that have not responded to medical measures. Repair of reducible hiatal hernia with tightening of the hiatus, or a gastroplasty type of operation for a fixed hiatal hernia, often substantially diminishes the need for further dilatation.

Dysphagia

Neoplastic dysphagia

Curative resection is the best means of treating carcinoma of the oesophagus or upper stomach causing dysphagia. In many patients, however, this is contraindicated by the presence of metastases or by the patient's poor general health, and palliative intubation with the Mousseau-Barbin or Celestin tube offers the only means of relieving distressing dysphagia and improving nutrition. In the past such intubation has been done by laparotomy and pull-through. This carries an immediate mortality of 25% and oral intubation under endoscopic control offers the advantages of relative safety and simplicity. The tube can be slid down the rigid oesophagoscope over a filiform bougie passed through the stricture. Today, however, fibreoptic endoscopic placement offers the most satisfactory method. After dilatation of the narrowing using the Eder-Puestow dilators in the same way as for peptic stricture, a Celestin tube cut to appropriate length and mounted on an introducer is passed along the Puestow guidewire until its position is satisfactory as judged by radiological screening. Most patients can take a semisolid diet within two days and can be discharged from hospital often on the third day. Particular attention must be given to careful mastication, and meals should be taken with fizzy drinks that help to prevent blockage of the tube.

Nutritional improvement often follows successful intubation, and squamous growths can be treated by radiotherapy with the tube in position. Rarely, the improvement in their general condition may be such that surgical resection of the growth may be reconsidered in patients previously too weak to withstand operation.

Gall stones

IAN A D BOUCHIER

In the 100 years after the first operation on the gall bladder by John Stough Bobbs cholecystectomy became the accepted method of treating cholelithiasis. The recent introduction of an agent that can safely dissolve gall stones and new advances in fibreoptic instruments have added new dimensions to managing this common and economically important disease. The doctor can now offer several therapeutic options to the patient with gall stones, and while this has enhanced the scope for manoeuvre it has created new and novel difficulties in decision making.

DIAGNOSIS

Gall stones may present in various ways. The most common and characteristic is either acute cholecystitis or obstruction of the common bile duct. Only 5% of patients with acute cholecystitis do not have coexistent gall stones. Less commonly stones may rupture into the bowel, obstruct the terminal ileum, or cause pancreatitis. Gall stones and cancer of the gall bladder may coexist. A few patients with acute cholecystitis may be icteric in the absence of choledocholithiasis but most patients with gall stones who are jaundiced will have a stone obstructing the common bile duct. Cholangitis is diagnosed when, in addition to the cholestasis, there are chills, fever, and pain and tenderness in the right upper quadrant. Flatulence, intolerance to fatty food, and vague right upper quadrant and epigastric pain are often ascribed to gall stones and chronic cholecystitis. Such complaints, however, are as often as not related to other common gastrointestinal disorders, and one of the major difficulties for the doctor is to decide what treatment to offer patients with gall stones who present with these symptoms.

Since only 15% of gall stones are radio-opaque a plain abdominal radiograph is often unhelpful. Oral cholecystography is the basic diagnostic tool, but if obstruction of the bile duct is suspected intravenous cholangiography, endoscopic retrograde cholangiopancreatography, percutaneous transhepatic cholangiography, and ultrasonic scanning may all be useful.

GALL STONES IN THE GALL BLADDER

Gall stones and acute cholecystitis are an indication for cholecystectomy, which is the most frequent major abdominal operation performed in Britain. The gall bladder is removed via a vertical paramedian incision or a subcostal incision, which is favoured in obese patients with a wide costal angle. Because choledocholithiasis occurs in some 10–15% of patients with gall-bladder stones it is generally accepted that operative cholangiography must be undertaken as a routine in all patients undergoing operation for gall stones. With experience the procedure adds little more than five minutes to the operating time and may be performed via a cannula in the cystic duct or by direct needle puncture of the common bile duct. Thus surgeons undertaking gall-bladder surgery must be capable of using the technique, and adequate radiographic facilities must be available in all operating theatres. The routine use of operative cholangiography has the advantage of reducing unnecessary bile-duct explorations; of diagnosing gall stones that would otherwise have been overlooked by palpation, thereby reducing the number of residual gall stones in the common bile duct; and of revealing unsuspected disease. The criticism that the procedure is accompanied by an increased morbidity is not convincing when the many benefits from operative cholangiography are considered.

While debate continues over the timing of the cholecystectomy in acute calculous cholecystitis, increasingly the consensus is moving towards early operation. On admission the patient is given such medical support as is appropriate. Analgesics recommended include morphine, pethidine, and pentazocine, the latter having the theoretical advantage that it does not raise biliary pressure. Intravenous fluids are given if the patient is vomiting, and an adequate urinary flow is maintained; it is seldom necessary to use a nasogastric tube. Appropriate treatment is given for associated cardiac or pulmonary disease. There is no evidence that anticholinergic agents are useful.

The rational use of antibiotics in acute cholecystitis remains controversial. Only half the patients coming to operation have infected bile, when various aerobic and anaerobic organisms may be cultured. The positive yield of bacteria increases if there is cystic duct obstruction or cholangitis. There is a correlation between the incidence of positive bile cultures and the frequency of wound infection, intra-abdominal sepsis, and the mortality rate. The choice of antibiotic may be governed by either the degree to which it is concentrated in the bile or the probable bacterial sensitivity. Unfortunately it seems that when there is liver dysfunction or obstruction of the cystic or common bile duct therapeutic levels of the antibiotic are unlikely to be achieved in the bile. Recommended antibiotics include parenteral cephaloridine (2–4 g daily), gentamicin (2–4 mg/kg/day), ampicillin (4 g daily), and tetracycline (2–4 g daily). Recent evidence, however, suggests that most organisms isolated from the biliary tract are not susceptible to ampicillin and tetracycline. Some authorities recommend using a Gram stain on uncentrifuged bile obtained at cholecystectomy as an aid to the choice of antibiotics, thereby avoiding unnecessary antibiotic prophylaxis.

Each patient will have to be considered individually, but generally the following recommendations may be made: no antibiotics are required for the average patient with acute gall-bladder inflammation; antibiotics are given if the illness is of more than four days' duration, if the clinical condition is deteriorating, or if there is any evidence of perforation, general peritonitis, or cholangitis.

Over 90% of patients improve after admission and may be operated on within five to 10 days. At this stage the predominant pathological features are oedema and congestion, which may even enhance the ease of dissection. Thereafter organisation and fibrosis become more prominent, making the procedure more difficult, so that an elective operation two to three months later may be no easier than if undertaken in the first 14 days. The advantage of the earlier operation is that there is a saving of time for the patient, whose illness is restricted to a single hospital admission. There is no difference in the mortality and morbidity figures when early and delayed operations are compared.

An emergency operation on the biliary tract is seldom needed because the average patient is not critically ill, but for the patient who is highly toxic or has a perforation, spreading infection, or severe cholangitis it will be necessary. In such cases a cholecystectomy may not be possible, and the wiser decision is to undertake a cholecystostomy. In this way the gall stones may be removed; but they will reform unless the gall bladder is removed later. Cholecystostomy is inadequate in the presence of acute cholangitis.

Gall-bladder disease in the elderly

Whereas the mortality among patients under the age of 50 undergoing cholecystectomy is less than 1%, it rises to nearly 3% in patients between 50 and 65 and approaches 8% in geriatric patients. Elderly patients tolerate emergency operations on the biliary tract poorly, and unfortunately it is in this group that most perforated or gangrenous gall bladders are found. A cholecystostomy may often be the most advantageous operation in the aged because it can be performed rapidly through a small incision and under a local anaesthetic if necessary. On recovery a cholangiogram is needed. If the biliary tree is normal there is no need for a further operation; if the gall bladder is not filled or stones are seen either in the gall bladder or in the duct system a cholecystectomy is warranted provided that the patient's general health is satisfactory.

Dissolution treatment

Great advances have been made in understanding the many factors concerned in the formation of gall stones. About 10% of gall stones from Western communities are composed purely of cholesterol, and

80% of the remainder contain at least 70% cholesterol. The outstanding biochemical abnormality in these patients is the secretion of hepatic bile that is saturated or supersaturated with cholesterol. At least two factors are responsible: the increased secretion of biliary cholesterol, and reduced secretion of bile acids in bile associated with a smaller than normal bile-acid pool. The initial observations by J L Thistle and L J Schoenfield, of the Mayo Clinic, that taking by mouth the primary bile acid chenodeoxycholic acid caused saturated hepatic bile to become unsaturated started an extensive study of chenodeoxycholic acid as a method of dissolving gall stones. Furthermore, it stimulated the search for other agents that might influence cholesterol output in bile.

Metabolism of chenodeoxycholic acid—Chenodeoxycholic acid (3α,7α-dihydroxy-5β-cholanic acid) is a primary bile acid derived semi-synthetically from animal bile and is similar to that produced normally in the human liver. It is absorbed to some extent by passive nonionic diffusion in the jejunum but the major absorption occurs in the distal ileum, where an active transport system ensures the conservation of free and conjugated bile acids. After returning to the liver, chenodeoxycholic acid is excreted in the bile, having been conjugated to glycine and taurine. Under the influence of intestinal bacteria, free and conjugated chenodeoxycholic acid undergoes 7α-dehydroxylation to the secondary bile acid lithocholic acid, which is either excreted in the stool or re-absorbed and returns via the portal circulation to the liver. There it is conjugated and most is additionally sulphated at the 3 position. The sulphated compounds are water-soluble, and thus once excreted in the bile they have a decidedly decreased intestinal absorption compared with the free and conjugated (but not sulphated) bile acid. In this way little lithocholic acid is retained in the body, which has important implications for hepatotoxicity.

Dose and selection of patients—Chenodeoxycholic acid is given as a gelatin capsule of 250 mg of the free bile acid. The optimal dose remains to be determined but doses used have ranged from 1·5 to 4·5 g daily; 10–15 mg/kg/day is probably adequate for the average patient. Attempts are being made to define a minimal effective dose. Available information indicates that chenodeoxycholic acid is effective only in patients who have radiolucent gall stones and functioning gall bladders; it is these patients who may be recommended for dissolution treatment. The indications for chenodeoxycholic acid treatment need defining. Some users have used the drug only for those patients who have been rejected by the surgeon as unfit for operation or for patients who have refused surgery; others have widened the scope for dissolution treatment and offered it to relatively fit patients with minimal symptoms. The current recommendation is that the agent should not be used in women of childbearing age. It usually takes between six and 24 months to dissolve gall stones, though multiple small stones respond more rapidly than a single large stone. Hence it is normally inappropriate to offer treatment to patients who have severe symptoms attributable to the gall stones or who are icteric. Chenodeoxycholic acid is currently under trial in several centres in Britain and is not yet available commercially.

Mode of action—Several mechanisms have been proposed to explain the action of chenodeoxycholic acid. The most favoured one is that it may reduce the output of cholesterol secreted into the bile. The hepatic synthesis of cholesterol is regulated by the microsomal enzyme 3-hydroxy-3-methylglutaryl-coenzyme A (HMG-CoA) reductase, while the rate-limiting enzyme for bile acid synthesis from cholesterol is 7α-hydroxylase. Chenodeoxycholic acid is believed to inhibit HMG-CoA reductase to a greater extent than it inhibits bile-acid synthesis, hence the reduction in biliary cholesterol secretion by the liver. Probably of secondary importance is the expansion in the bile-acid pool accompanying taking exogenous chenodeoxycholic acid.

Evaluation of treatment—Treatment may be evaluated in two ways. A cholecystogram may be taken at about six-monthly intervals until the stones have dissolved. Additionally, samples of bile obtained by duodenal drainage may be measured for the degree of cholesterol saturation. It has been argued that the effective dose of chenodeoxycholic acid is one that causes the bile to become unsaturated with cholesterol; but some users have reported that the measurement of cholesterol saturation in bile does not always predict effective response to the bile acid.

Response to treatment—Opinions differ on how effective chenodeoxycholic acid is when given to apparently suitable patients. Most users find that successful dissolution can be achieved in over half the patients, and at least one group has suggested that the success rate will approach 100% if bile can be maintained unsaturated with cholesterol. The bile acid should be continued for at least three to six months after stones are no longer identified on the cholecystogram. Unfortunately some patients return to excreting saturated bile after chenodeoxycholic acid is discontinued and the gall stones recur. It is still uncertain what should be the long-term management of patients who have responded to dissolution treatment: should the drug be discontinued or should the patient continue to take a smaller dose that is just enough to maintain the bile in an unsaturated state?

Side effects—Chenodeoxycholic acid has proved to be remarkably safe in clinical practice. Minor diarrhoea, which is caused by the colonic secretion of water and electrolytes induced by the free bile acid, is readily reversed by reducing the dose. A transient mild (less than twice normal) increase in hepatic transaminases or alkaline phosphatase or both may occur in the initial months of treatment but resolves spontaneously and is not an indication to stop treatment. So far no meaningful changes have been reported in the cholesterol pool size. Extensive liver biopsy studies with comparison before and after chenodeoxycholic acid treatment have failed to show any appreciable morphological changes. Electron microscopical studies have shown a slight increase in Ito cells, the significance of which is not apparent. These observations are both interesting and reassuring because of the recognised hepatotoxic effects of lithocholic acid and the severe liver damage that has been seen under certain conditions in animals fed chenodeoxycholic acid. The probable reason for the difference between the human and animal results is the sulphation of lithocholates, thereby preventing the accumulation of this bile acid in the enterohepatic circulation.

Other agents used to dissolve gall stones—No other drug is as effective as chenodeoxycholic acid in dissolving gall stones. Cholic acid has been evaluated and is ineffective, probably because it has a different effect on the rate-limiting enzymes of cholesterol and bile-acid synthesis. The use of lecithin remains controversial. Phenobarbitone has been tried but it appears to be ineffective when used on its own, and there is no advantage in combining it with chenodeoxycholic acid. Ursodeoxycholic acid, the 7β epimer of chenodeoxycholic acid, increases in the bile of patients given chenodeoxycholic acid. It has been suggested that this metabolite might dissolve gall stones but there are insufficient supportive data.

Influence of diet

There is no acceptable evidence that any particular diet influences gall-bladder or gall-stone disease. A low-fat diet is often prescribed but has not been evaluated satisfactorily. It remains to be determined how much beneficial effect such a diet has either on symptoms or on the underlying disorder of hepatic metabolism or the gall-bladder function and, if any effect is present, whether it is due to the low fat content of the diet, a reduction in calories, or a concomitant increase in the dietary fibre content.

The silent stone

The management of the silent gall stone remains one of the most vexed and controversial issues in biliary tract disease. Should silent stones be removed? The answer is often Yes, and in support the excellent study of A Wenckert and B Robertson is quoted, which showed that 35% of patients with gall stones followed up for 11 years developed complications. It must be emphasised, however, that the patients under study did not have silent stones: they had all presented with some feature of gall-stone disease. By definition a silent stone should be completely asymptomatic, and it is impossible to see how these might be diagnosed during life. Evidence from necropsy data suggests that truly silent gall stones are not uncommon. The treatment of the silent stone is uncertain, with arguments favouring cholecystectomy contrasting with the attitude that the stones should be left alone. My personal prejudice is for the latter approach. It would be comforting to think that chenodeoxycholic acid might be used for these patients and, indeed, it may, except that so many silent stones are radio-opaque that have been discovered by chance on plain radiographs of the abdomen, and these stones are unsuitable for dissolution treatment.

STONES IN COMMON BILE DUCT

The presence of stones in the common bile duct is generally an indication for laparotomy, cholecystectomy, and exploration of the common bile duct. Preoperative preparation includes giving parenteral vitamin K if jaundice is present (5–10 mg daily for three days) and antibiotic cover. The intravenous administration of 500 ml of a 10% solution of mannitol one hour before the operation helps to reduce the risk of the patient with deep jaundice developing acute renal failure. An operative cholangiogram is always recommended. The usual procedure is a supraduodenal choledochotomy with T-tube drainage. The T tube is left for seven to 10 days, and before removal a cholangiogram is usually obtained. A transduodenal sphincterotomy may be attempted if the gall stones are impacted at the lower end of the common bile duct, and in such cases T-tube drainage may be unnecessary.

About 2% of patients who have undergone choledochotomy subsequently have residual bile-duct stones. Many of these patients are unsuitable for further surgery, and other methods have been proposed for dealing with the stones. If the T tube is still present it may be possible to pass, under radiological control, a urethral stone basket. Another method that has received encouraging reports is the infusion, via the T tube, of 100 M sodium cholate at a rate of 30 ml hourly for 10 days. It is usually necessary to take cholestyramine by mouth (6–12 g daily) to reduce any diarrhoea. An infusion of heparin (25 000 units eight-hourly) via the tube has also been recommended. None of these methods has been subjected to an adequate clinical trial, and present information indicates that irrigation of the common bile duct with a simple saline washout might be just as effective.

A method of great interest is the removal of gall stones by means of a fibreoptic duodenoscope suitably modified and equipped to perform a papillotomy. At a later date the endoscope is passed again and the stone may be removed using a Dormia catheter. This technique calls for great skill and at present is suitable only for relatively small stones.

If the gall stone is discovered after the T tube has been removed oral chenodeoxycholic acid treatment may be attempted; there is no point in using this agent to infuse down a T tube because cholic acid is as effective. Favourable results have been reported in some patients, who have had fewer episodes of cholangitis and ultimate stone dissolution; but many patients have not responded.

It needs to be emphasised that the accepted treatment for choledocholithiasis is surgical removal. All other methods are to some extent under trial and are mainly relevant to those patients who are unsuitable for further surgery.

THE FUTURE

The future must lie with the development and better understanding of dissolution treatment. It is necessary to predict more accurately which patients will respond to treatment. The correct dose of chenodeoxycholic acid needs definition, and clear indications are needed for deciding when to stop treatment both in responders and in non-responders. Of great importance is the development of a rational programme for the management of those patients whose gall stones have dissolved. For this the suggestion that a high intake of dietary fibre might favourably influence cholesterol solubility in bile is relevant. Perhaps the most important lesson to be learnt from chenodeoxycholic acid treatment is that bile composition can be manipulated to render it unsaturated with cholesterol. This has important implications for preventing gall stones. Although saturated bile is only one aspect of the complicated mechanism for gall-stone formation, gall stones might possibly be prevented by influencing bile composition. Probably drug treatment will not be the solution. The promising work with fibre-rich diets points the way, and it may well be that the ultimate solution to gall-stone disease will be the rational use of specific diets.

I thank the Medical Research Council and Weddell Pharmaceuticals for support.

FURTHER READING

Bell, G D, *Gut*, 1974, **15**, 913.
Bouchier, I A D, *Gallstones in Modern Trends in Gastroenterology*, ed A E Read. London, Butterworths, 1975.
Dawson, J L, *Clinics in Gastroenterology*, 1973, **2**, 85.
Kune, G A, *Current Practice of Biliary Surgery*. Boston, Little Brown, 1972.
Schein, C J, *Acute Cholecystitis*. New York, Harper and Row, 1972.
Schoenfield, L J, *Gastroenterology*, 1974, **67**, 725.

Jaundice

IAIN M MURRAY-LYON, KEITH REYNOLDS

A rational approach to treating the patient with jaundice depends on accurate diagnosis. Despite a wide range of new laboratory tests and diagnostic techniques the emphasis still lies initially on careful history taking and physical examination. All too often the patient with drug-induced jaundice undergoes unnecessary laparotomy because the appropriate questions are not asked and an adequate history of alcohol consumption is rarely taken. In other patients the tell-tale physical stigmata of chronic liver disease such as spider naevi and palmar erythema are overlooked.

CURRENT DIAGNOSTIC METHODS

The battery of standard liver function tests generally used in Britain (serum bilirubin, aspartate and alanine aminotransferases, and alkaline phosphatase) may point clearly to viral hepatitis (high transaminases of 1000 IU/l or more and a modest rise in alkaline phosphatase) or to an obstructive cause, when the alkaline phosphatase is 30 King-Armstrong units or more with a smaller rise in transaminases; but often the pattern of change is indeterminate. Further biochemical investigation is seldom rewarding except in the rare instances when specific plasma protein assays may indicate a specific diagnosis—for instance, low values of caeruloplasmin in Wilson's disease, greatly raised level of α-fetoprotein in primary liver cancer, and deficiency of α_1-antitrypsin. A rise in the serum bilirubin concentration with otherwise normal liver function is often found now that automated biochemical screening is widely established. In the absence of notable haemolysis (anaemia and raised reticulocyte count) this rise is often caused by constitutional hyperbilirubinaemia (Gilbert's syndrome), and the bilirubin is predominantly unconjugated (indirect reacting). The intravenous nicotinic acid test[1] is proving useful in establishing the diagnosis and often obviates the need for liver biopsy.

Detection of hepatitis B surface antigen (HBsAg) in the serum suggests that the jaundice is caused either by acute type B hepatitis or by chronic liver disease associated with persistence of the virus. We now know that many viruses may cause acute hepatitis, and techniques for diagnosing infection with cytomegalovirus and the EB virus of glandular fever are readily available. The presence of autoantibodies to smooth muscle, nuclei, or mitochondria point to one of the autoimmune liver disorders, such as active chronic hepatitis or primary biliary cirrhosis. Secondary syphilis as the cause of jaundice should never be forgotten, and appropriate serological testing is never out of place.

Liver scanning has become established as a safe and useful method of diagnosis, particularly for focal lesions such as metastatic deposits and abscesses. The scanning material usually used is ^{99m}Tc-sulphur colloid, which is taken up by the Kupffer cells. Further information about the nature of any abnormality may be gained by using other scanning materials such as ^{75}Se-selenomethionine (for primary hepatocellular carcinoma) or ^{67}Ga-citrate (for tumour or abscess), and grey-scale ultrasound,[2] which is not yet available in all centres, adds further information about the consistency of focal hepatic lesions, and because of its high resolution it may show up dilated intrahepatic bile ducts. The EMI body scanner, when it becomes generally available may add further important information about the disposition of the abdominal organs and prove valuable in diagnosing carcinoma of the pancreas, which is a common cause of obstructive jaundice in middle-aged and elderly patients.

For many years needle biopsy of the liver has been valuable in the differential diagnosis of the jaundiced patient, and it is a safe procedure in experienced hands. It has recently been shown that infusions of clotting-factor concentrates or fresh-frozen plasma may allow biopsy specimens to be taken even when the prothrombin time is greatly prolonged.[3] The diagnostic accuracy is increased when the specimen is taken under direct vision from abnormal areas in the liver at laparoscopy. Much experience is needed for accurate interpretation of needle biopsy findings, but, unlike the case with renal tissue, the use of immunofluorescence techniques and electron microscopy has not yet contributed appreciably to clinical practice.

Techniques for visualising the biliary tree in cases of suspected extrahepatic obstructive jaundice have improved greatly in recent years. Intravenous cholangiography is seldom successful when the serum bilirubin is greater than 34 μmol/l (2 mg/100 ml) but dye can be injected directly into the dilated intrahepatic biliary tree (percutaneous transhepatic cholangiography). The development in Japan of a new fine flexible (skinny) needle[4] has made the procedure safer, and allowed the outlining of the normal biliary tree. Because there is some risk of biliary peritonitis the investigation is best done with a surgical colleague, so that the latter can proceed to laparotomy on the same day if extrahepatic obstruction is found. Endoscopic retrograde cholangiopancreatography with the side-viewing fibreoptic panendoscope offers an alternative means of obtaining cholangiograms in the jaundiced patient. Pancreatograms may also show that the primary disease lies in the pancreas, usually a carcinoma but sometimes chronic pancreatitis. As this technique demands frequent practice and a high degree of expertise it is less readily applicable in smaller hospitals, where preoperative cholangiography is seldom needed. Plain films of the abdomen and chest should never be omitted, as they may hold vital information such as radio-opaque gall stones or metastatic deposits, and a barium meal (or better a double-contrast duodenogram) may show changes suggestive of carcinoma of the pancreas.

CURRENT TREATMENT

Viral hepatitis

The mainstay of treatment for viral hepatitis remains a nutritious diet and bed rest, although various clinical trials have failed to show that bed rest is beneficial. There is now increasing evidence that the use of corticosteroids may be harmful, especially in type B hepatitis (HBsAg-positive), as their use tends to lead to chronicity. During the recovery phase the traditional three to six months' embargo on alcohol remains in vogue, and careful follow-up with serial liver function tests is important to detect those cases (5–10%) in which chronic liver disease will develop. Transmission of hepatitis to family members and medical staff is unusual if conventional precautions are taken, but if there is any risk of parenteral inoculation a good degree of protection is given against type A hepatitis (HBsAg-negative) by an intramuscular injection of standard immunoglobulin (γ-globulin) and against type B hepatitis by specific high-titre anti-HBs immunoglobulin, which is now obtainable in limited amounts from the directors of the local public health laboratory service.

Fulminant hepatic failure

A few patients with viral hepatitis (especially type B) develop massive hepatic necrosis with a severe bleeding diathesis and coma. Other causes of this syndrome include overdoses with paracetamol, a hypersensitivity reaction to antituberculosis drugs, and multiple halothane anaesthetics. Detailed discussion of the management of these critically ill patients is beyond the scope of this article,[5] but they need intensive medical and nursing care with regular monitoring of all body functions. The blood sugar concentration is maintained by intravenous dextrose infusions, and lactulose or neomycin or both are given to combat the coma, which is thought to be caused at least partly by intestinal absorption of various toxins derived from bacterial breakdown of protein in the gut. Corticosteroids, although often used, have not been shown to be of benefit. The complications of the disease are legion, and artificial ventilation and renal dialysis are often needed. Because of the enormous capacity of the liver to regenerate, various liver-support systems have been developed in an attempt to buy enough time for recovery to occur. Exchange transfusion and pig-liver perfusion both enjoyed popularity for a time, but neither has been shown to improve the survival figures. Interest currently centres on artificial liver-support systems such as charcoal haemoperfusion and haemodialysis with new, large-pore membranes.[6] The mortality remains high at around 70–80% in patients who become comatose, but in those who do recover, liver regeneration restores the hepatic architecture to normal and cirrhosis does not develop.

Active chronic hepatitis

Several well-conducted trials have now put the treatment of active chronic hepatitis on a surer footing.[7] Corticosteroids improve liver function and also prolong survival, but at the cost of many serious side effects. Immunosuppressive treatment with azathioprine alone is ineffective. After initial control of the disease with large doses of corticosteroids the best current maintenance treatment regimen is prednisolone 5 mg twice a day with azathioprine 50 mg daily. Treatment usually needs to be continued for several years, and there is a high relapse rate after its withdrawal. Alternate-day prednisolone regimens that have proved successful in some other conditions have not yet been shown to be as good as daily treatment, and they cannot yet be recommended.

Careful follow-up of these cases is important, and the efficacy of treatment is best monitored by regular liver biopsy. If corticosteroid side effects are troublesome, penicillamine is a satisfactory but more toxic alternative drug for maintaining remission. Probably cases associated with persistence of the hepatitis B antigen are less responsive to treatment and tend to progress relentlessly towards cirrhosis.

Primary biliary cirrhosis

Patients should receive monthly intramuscular supplements of vitamins A, D, and K because of the malabsorption of fat-soluble vitamins. Pruritus is often distressing and may be controlled by the anion exchange resin cholestyramine. No treatment has yet been shown to alter the relentless progress of the disease. Corticosteroids are ineffective and hasten bone thinning, and a recent prospective controlled trial of azathioprine versus placebo failed to show any improvement in liver function values or survival, and progression to cirrhosis was unaffected.[8]

SOME SURGICAL CONSIDERATIONS

Jaundiced patients

In patients with extrahepatic obstructive jaundice bile stasis often leads to infection, and thus surgery may be complicated by bacteraemia and endotoxic shock. The syndrome of hypotension, worsening liver function, and renal failure (the hepatorenal syndrome) is a major cause of death in these patients. This has led to the use of forced diuresis with mannitol and intravenous antibiotics, starting before the operation.

Hypotension should be prevented at all costs, and oliguria is watched for by using an indwelling catheter. The central venous pressure should be continually monitored postoperatively. Routine monitoring of blood urea and serum electrolyte concentrations will pick up the early development of hypercatabolic renal failure. The routine use of such measures has greatly reduced the morbidity and mortality in surgical patients with obstructive jaundice.

Peroperative cholangiography

The necessity for routine peroperative cholangiography in patients with jaundice cannot be overemphasised. Apart from the obvious benefit of showing stones and the site (and often the nature) of strictures of the common bile duct the routine use of the image intensifier and television screen allows the kinetics of the duct to be studied. This is of particular value in cases where a dilated duct is found and no primary intraductal disorder is shown on routine cholangiography performed at the time of operation. Such cases, often previously labelled as biliary dyskinesia, can often be shown to have stenosis or stricture at the level of the papilla of Vater. In specialised centres pressure profiles of the common duct, measured with a fine-bore cardiac catheter, may be useful when combined with cholangiography.

Acute cholecystitis

Most surgeons prefer to manage patients with acute cholecystitis conservatively by bed rest, analgesics, and oral or intravenous fluids according to the severity of the attack. The need for antibiotics is debatable, but associated cholangitis or the development of acute pancreatitis or bacteraemia is an absolute indication for their use. In these circumstances careful observation is important as surgical intervention may be necessary.

Spreading or generalised peritonitis may be either biliary or purulent in origin, and is usually secondary to necrosis of the gall bladder fundus and an absolute indication for laparotomy. In these cases simple drainage of the peritoneal cavity with a cholecystostomy may be life saving, particularly if the region of the common bile duct and porta hepatis is surrounded by a dense inflammatory mass (phlegmon) secondary to antibiotic treatment.

What should the surgeon do when he finds acute cholecystitis at emergency laparotomy? In the elderly and frail or obviously toxic and ill patients a large mucocele or empyaema is usually found, and a simple cholecystostomy—removal of the impacted stone followed by the insertion of a Foley catheter and external biliary fistula—may be life saving. An elective cholecystectomy may be performed later. In younger and fitter patients where the anatomy of the cystic triangle is clearly and easily defined cholecystectomy is the operation of choice. The role of emergency peroperative cholangiography in these cases is debatable, but in suppurative cholangitis it is best to drain the common duct via a T tube.

Residual ductal stones

The residual ductal stone is found in two different circumstances: when the stone has been left at the previous exploration of the duct and a T tube is still in situ, and when a patient subsequently presents with obstructive jaundice, often many months after surgery.

In the first condition, if the stone is small or fragmented perfusion of the T tube with heparinised saline or sodium cholate with concomitant use of antispasmodics may be tried.[9] If a surgical approach is used peroperative cholangiography is essential, and choledochograms after removal of the stone are necessary to exclude associated conditions of the lower end of the common bile duct. Recently stones at the lower end of the common bile duct have been successfully removed by endoscopic papillotomy with a side-viewing gastroscope.[10] When the residual stone presents later and only slight jaundice allows the stone to be clearly seen on preoperative intravenous cholangiography, the transduodenal approach to the bile duct with sphincteroplasty is the obvious method of choice when dense adhesions surround the previous operative site. Peroperative intravenous aprotinin (Trasylol) minimises the development of clinical pancreatitis, although postoperatively the serum amylase rises. Endoscopic papillotomy may also be tried in specialist centres. With severe obstructive jaundice the site of obstruction should be shown by either retrograde cholangiopancreatography or percutaneous transhepatic cholangiography just before laparotomy. The transduodenal approach is ideal for stone impacted in the lower end of the common bile duct, but in high-risk cases with severe jaundice and septicaemia simple T-tube drainage of the bile duct is indicated with forced diuresis and appropriate antibiotic cover. Elective surgery may be undertaken later after control of infection and T-tube cholangiography.

REFERENCES

1 Fromke, V L, and Miller, D, *Medicine*, 1972, **51,** 451.
2 Taylor, K J W, *et al, Journal of Clinical Ultrasound*, 1973, **1,** 284.
3 Gazzard, B G, *et al, Gut*, 1975, **16,** 621.
4 Okuda, K, *et al, American Journal of Digestive Diseases*, 1974, **19,** 21.

[5] Murray-Lyon, I M, and Trewby, P, in *Recent Advances in Intensive Therapy*, ed I M Ledingham, vol 1. Edinburgh, Churchill Livingstone, 1976. In press.
[6] Williams, R, and Murray-Lyon, I M, *Artificial Liver Support*. Tunbridge Wells, Pitman Medical, 1975.
[7] Summerskill, W H J, *et al*, *Gut*, 1975, **16,** 876.
[8] Heathcote, J, Ross, A, and Sherlock, S, *Gastroenterology*, 1976, **70,** 656.
[9] Bell, G D, *Gut*, 1974, **15,** 913.
[10] Classen, M, and Safrany, L, *British Medical Journal*, 1975, **4,** 371.

Drug jaundice

ALEX PATON

There may be no drug (or chemical) that is entirely free from the risk of causing liver damage, so central is the liver's role in the metabolism of foreign substances. The metabolic processes are diverse and complex, and disposal of a drug is not necessarily synonymous with detoxication, since in some cases—paracetamol, for example—a more toxic substance may be produced. Fortunately, however, the liver has considerable reserve, so that the risk of damage is dependent either on overwhelming doses of drugs (causing hepatic necrosis) or on a relatively uncommon individual hypersensitivity, which may be due to defective enzyme systems and is at present usually unpredictable.

Local environmental factors are also important. Blood flow to the liver, its oxygenation, the state of enzyme activity—for example, enzyme induction—and the competing claims of other substances, such as alcohol and steroid hormones, for metabolic pathways will all affect the response to a drug.

The detailed classification of drug damage can be found in standard texts. Since jaundice is the usual adverse reaction to drugs, I propose to concentrate on the two syndromes of hepatitis and cholestasis. Generally, the reaction to a particular drug is confined to one or other of these, but a few drugs may apparently cause both types of jaundice: these are indicated in the table, which lists only the better-known examples of drugs associated with jaundice. I shall also consider briefly the important question whether drug damage can lead to chronic liver disease.

Drugs causing hepatitis or cholestasis or both

Hepatitis	Cholestasis
Monoamine oxidase inhibitors	Phenothiazines
Antidepressants	Benzodiazepines
Anaesthetic agents including halothane	Antihistamines†
Anticonvulsants	Oral hypoglycaemic agents
Barbiturates*	Diuretics†
Antituberculous drugs*	Antithyroid agents
Sulphonamides*	Nitrofurantoin
Anti-inflammatory drugs	Oestrogens
Appetite suppressants	Progestogens
Beta-blockers	
Methyldopa*	

* May also cause cholestasis.
† May also cause hepatitis.

HEPATITIS

The clinical picture of drug hepatitis mimics that of other types of hepatitis, though it is sometimes possible to recognise minor differences. The interval between prodromal symptoms and jaundice, and their prominence, is often less than in viral hepatitis, and features of hypersensitivity may be pronounced. Abdominal pain is sometimes particularly severe and is a bad prognostic sign. The course of the illness varies from a minor nuisance to death within a few days from acute hepatic necrosis.

The mechanism of drug hepatitis is unknown but is most likely to be caused by hypersensitivity. The similarity to viral hepatitis has led some people to the view that a latent virus is stimulated by the drug. Nevertheless, spread from person to person is unknown, second attacks have occurred on re-exposure, and the mortality from drug hepatitis (which may reach 30% in certain cases) is considerably higher than that of viral hepatitis. Moreover, jaundice may be predicted with chemically related compounds, as in the case of monoamine-oxidase inhibitors and anti-inflammatory drugs. None of these arguments is conclusive, however, and the answer must await isolation of the viruses or a specific test for drug sensitivity. The practice of monitoring the effect on the liver by measuring serum aminotransferase levels may be misleading since rises often occur at the beginning of treatment, possibly owing to enzyme induction. Once hepatitis is suspected the only safe course is to stop the drug and not to use it again.

Such a practice may lead to difficult problems in management as in the case of antituberculous agents, all of which, except streptomycin and possibly some of the newer drugs (though caution is essential with drugs that have not been in use for long), may cause jaundice. Intermittent use of a drug may increase the risk of hepatitis, an example being the jaundice that follows repeated exposure to halothane. This is not the place to discuss the halothane controversy, but, while most cases of postoperative jaundice in which halothane has been given can be explained on other grounds, there is a small residue in which no factor other than halothane can be implicated.

Most drug hepatitis is not dose-related. This is not so with paracetamol, which together with carbon tetrachloride and a few other poisons is a direct hepatotoxin causing acute necrosis. Doses above 15 g are invariably accompanied by liver cell damage, and in severe cases the kidneys, gastrointestinal tract, and brain may also be implicated, a feature of hepatic necrosis from whatever cause. Acute necrosis has also followed inhalation of solvents by glue sniffers.

CHOLESTASIS

The second type of reaction resembles obstructive jaundice both clinically and biochemically. It is caused by intrahepatic cholestasis and cannot be distinguished from mechanical obstruction, although severe pruritis is more likely to be caused by drug cholestasis.

Cholestatic jaundice is a hypersensitivity reaction, so its occurrence and frequency are unpredictable. It may occur after a few doses of a drug or after years of treatment; vanish or persist after stopping the drug; disappear while treatment continues; and does not always recur when the offending drug is given again. If jaundice occurs with one member of a group of drugs—for example, phenothiazines—it is likely with others. Once obstruction is complete it may take months for jaundice to subside, so that the diagnosis is questioned and operation may be undertaken, with disastrous results. In spite of the equivocal nature of drug cholestasis and its generally benign nature, the wisest course is to stop the drug and avoid its use in the future.

It is usual to distinguish two groups of cholestatic drugs. The first are those such as the phenothiazines in which histological changes are characterised not only by cholestasis but also by spotty "degenerative" changes in liver cells and portal tract infiltration, especially with eosinophils. The presence of liver cell damage may account for the fact that fatalities have occurred in this group. By contrast, the second group, in which bile stasis only is seen on liver biopsy, appear to be relatively benign. This so-called "steroid jaundice" was first recognised with methyltestosterone and has since come to be associated with anabolic steroids and the pill. It is to some extent dose-related, and my impression is that its frequency has fallen considerably since the introduction of the "low dose" pill. There is, however, an element of hypersensitivity, since it occurs in families and in women who develop itching and jaundice during pregnancy. If jaundice is going to result from the pill it will do so during the first few cycles. Possibly other cholestatic drugs should be avoided in such women: one of my patients developed an identical reaction to diazepam some years after pill jaundice.

CHRONIC LIVER DISEASE

As already mentioned, some drugs produce a variety of liver damage. This is particularly true of methyldopa and the fact that it and other drugs—for example, oxyphenisatin—have been associated with chronic active hepatitis raises the important question whether drugs can cause cirrhosis. A few cases of biliary cirrhosis have followed the use of phenothiazines, and it has been suggested that primary biliary cirrhosis —a disease of unknown aetiology—might result from the habit among middle-aged women of taking rejuvenating medicines containing small amounts of testosterone. The pill can occasionally cause hepatic vein thrombosis, with severe abdominal pain; a tender, swollen liver; ascites;

and the rapid development of portal hypertension, which if not quickly fatal results in cirrhosis. Hepatic fibrosis and cirrhosis sometimes follow methotrexate treatment of psoriasis and have been reported with other cytotoxic drugs in the treatment of malignant lymphoma.

All these are rather special and isolated examples. There is as yet no evidence that drug usage in general can lead to cirrhosis. Nevertheless, repeated doses of drugs known to be associated with liver damage over a long period could possibly lead to cirrhosis in a susceptible person, in much the same way that alcohol results in cirrhosis. A third of the patients in this country have cryptogenic cirrhosis, and a study of their drug-taking habits might be worthwhile.

Significance of persistent HBs antigenaemia

IAN WOOLF, ROGER WILLIAMS

It is well established that the presence of hepatitis B surface antigen (HBsAg) in blood indicates infection with the hepatitis B virus. HBsAg constitutes the surface of the 42-nm Dane particle, which may well be the complete virus, and is also the antigen of the 20-nm spherical and tubular forms that exist, probably as a result of overproduction of this surface component. HBsAg may be detected during the incubation period of acute hepatitis type B, and in cases that follow the usual course to complete recovery it has invariably disappeared three months after the onset of the illness. Subsequently the corresponding antibody (anti-HBs) may be detected, which persists for months or even years. The core of the Dane particle contains a second antigen, hepatitis B core antigen (HBcAg), which has also been found in the nuclei of infected hepatocytes. Free HBcAg has not been detected in blood but its antibody (HBcAb) appears during or just before the onset of acute hepatitis type B and probably persists indefinitely.

WHO ARE HBSAG-POSITIVE?

HBsAg, however, does persist in the serum in certain conditions. A few patients, for example, may remain HBsAg-positive after acute hepatitis type B. This occurred in 11 out of 253 such patients (4·3%) in Copenhagen, and all showed evidence of chronic liver disease.[1] In haemodialysis and renal transplantation units infection with hepatitis B virus is often followed by persistent HBs antigenaemia. This may result from an impaired immune response to hepatitis B viral antigens through either the toxic effect of renal failure in the dialysis patients or treatment with immunosuppressives in those patients who have had transplants. This persistent HBs antigenaemia is often although not invariably associated with the development of a chronic hepatitis.

Some patients with evidence of chronic liver disease, with or without a history of hepatitis, will be HBsAg-positive. The proportion will depend on the population studied. Thus with the use of a sensitive radioimmunoassay technique only 13% of a series of British-born patients with chronic active hepatitis were shown to be HBsAg-positive, whereas among a similar group of patients originating from either the Mediterranean area or the Middle East the proportion was 60%.[2]

Finally, HBsAg may be present persistently in asymptomatic people without a history of hepatitis or signs of chronic liver disease. Such people are usually referred to as "carriers". Carriers are common in institutions for the mentally handicapped, particularly among adults committed since childhood, but they also exist in the normal population. For instance, the prevalence of HBsAg among blood donors in Britain is about 1/1000. Higher rates (up to 1%) have been recorded in commercial blood donors in the USA, reflecting the high proportion of drug addicts and the low socioeconomic status of such donor populations, while rates of up to 6% have been recorded in parts of Africa.

HBSAG-POSITIVE CHRONIC LIVER DISEASE

Detailed investigations of HBsAg-positive blood donors have shown evidence of liver disease in some, particularly when many drug addicts have been included among the donors investigated. In a study in north-west England,[3] 40 out of 110 HBsAg-positive blood donors (36%), none of whom were parenteral drug users, showed abnormalities of liver function, particularly raised aminotransferase levels. In only six instances, however, did liver biopsy show a serious condition such as chronic aggressive hepatitis or cirrhosis, although further follow-up showed progression from persistent hepatitis to chronic aggressive hepatitis in two more. With a longer period of follow-up further evidence of progression may be found, but it is worth noting that the "healthy" carrier differs from the patient with HBsAg-positive chronic liver disease in several respects.

Firstly, there are notable differences in the distribution of both HBsAg and HBcAg in the liver. Intranuclear HBcAg may be found in many hepatocytes from patients with chronic liver disease but in few if any hepatocytes from healthy carriers. HBsAg, which is found in the cytoplasm, is present in less than 5% of hepatocytes in chronic liver disease and is scattered in random fashion throughout each lobule. In healthy carriers up to half the cells may contain HBsAg, which tends to occur in clumps or large sheets of affected hepatocytes. This accords with our understanding of the basic immunological defect in those carriers in whom no cellular immunity to HBsAg is detectable. This failure of immunity presumably allows the virus to exist in harmless symbiosis with its host, and direct cell-to-cell spread of virus may consequently occur. In HBsAg-positive chronic active hepatitis, on the other hand, cellular immunity to HBsAg is present. Infected hepatocytes with viral determinants on their surface are consequently destroyed, which accounts for the finding of comparatively few HBsAg-containing cells. Indeed, in one study on eight patients with this condition, HBsAg was never found on the liver cell surface but only in the cytoplasm, where it is presumably immune from attack. Similarly, the many infected cells that contain core antigen in their nuclei, but which have not yet synthesised the coat protein, cannot be destroyed.

The absence of core particles from the nuclei of hepatocytes from healthy carriers is mirrored by an absence of Dane particles from the serum when examined with the electron microscope. Conversely, Dane particles are usually present in the serum of patients with HBsAg-positive chronic liver disease.

e Antigen—another antigen-antibody system in HBsAg-positive sera, but serologically distinct from HBsAg, was described in 1972[4] and designated "e." This e antigen-antibody system has provided another difference between the healthy carrier and the patient with HBsAg-positive chronic liver disease. e Antigen is not found in healthy carriers but is often present in patients with chronic liver disease, particularly those with chronic aggressive hepatitis. Some correlation between the detection of e antigen and the presence of Dane particles also exists. e Antigen may be associated with DNA polymerase, which is detectable in sera containing Dane particles.

DANGERS FROM HBSAG CARRIERS

From a public health point of view, the potential infectivity of the healthy carrier is of great importance. The HBsAg carrier has been described as "the leper of the 20th century," which, since his detection usually results from an act of altruism—namely, donating blood—is a cruel irony. Is this description justified? Clearly HBsAg-positive blood cannot be accepted for transfusion, but should further restrictions be placed on the activities of a carrier? It is certainly advisable to exclude such people from working in haemodialysis and renal transplantation units. Both patients and staff in these units should be tested regularly for HBsAg and those found to be positive treated in isolation. The institution of such a policy in Britain has led to the virtual elimination of type B hepatitis from these units. In other parts of the world the infection in renal units continues to be rife.

Nevertheless, despite the accumulating evidence for the non-parenteral transmission of hepatitis B virus as a major mode of spread, the possibility that healthy carriers may transmit infection remains debatable. Serological studies of the families and household contacts of patients with HBsAg-positive chronic liver disease have indicated that transmission of infection often occurs through intimate domestic and sexual contact. By contrast, in the families and household contacts of healthy carriers evidence of exposure to hepatitis B virus is rarely found. In a retrospective investigation in Sweden only two out of 16 long-term HBsAg carriers were implicated in cases of transfusion hepatitis, although all of them had previously donated much blood before their HBsAg state was discovered.[5] Furthermore, at the time of the investigation transfusion hepatitis was usually associated with the ay subtype of HBsAg, whereas most of the long-term carriers were of subtype ad, which was the predominant subtype of HBsAg associated with type B hepatitis in Sweden 20 years previously. Similarly, although transmission of hepatitis B from an HBsAg-positive mother to her newborn infant is a recognised hazard, it is much more likely to occur to the infant of a woman contracting type B hepatitis in the last trimester than to the child of a healthy carrier. In the Far East, where HBsAg is much more prevalent, transmission from asymptomatic carrier mothers to their infants is not uncommon, but when it does occur e antigen has been detected in the maternal serum, suggesting that these women are not truly healthy carriers.

There is little evidence that persistent HBsAg carriers concerned in medical care transmit hepatitis B. Alter *et al*[6] followed up 171 patients who were contacts of three healthy HBsAg carriers—two doctors and one nurse—for six to nine months. None of these patients developed type B hepatitis. A recent survey of dental surgeons at King's College Hospital, prompted by reports that the prevalence of HBsAg carriage in dentists was higher than in the general population, showed no evidence of transmission of hepatitis from an HBsAg-positive dentist to his patients. Although one such case has been reported, the dentist concerned was suffering from chronic liver disease. Thus apart from the special circumstances of renal dialysis units and blood transfusion laboratories, where the risk of hepatitis is great, there appears to be no justification for restricting the activities of a healthy HBsAg-positive health care worker unless he has been definitely implicated in an outbreak of hepatitis.

The detailed investigation of the apparently healthy carrier is important in two respects. Primarily it will permit the identification of occult chronic liver disease, which may need future treatment, at an early stage. Secondly, in most instances where no such abnormality is found, these people may be reassured that they are neither harbouring a serious illness nor are they a great danger to the health of others.

HEPATITIS B VACCINE

Finally, mention should be made of efforts to produce a hepatitis B vaccine. Since HBsAb is a protective antibody, vaccines containing HBsAg in a non-infectious form may prove valuable. Maupas *et al* have reported the results of a vaccination programme using a vaccine prepared from the sera of patients with persistent HBs antigenaemia that were free of Dane particles and negative for e antigen.[7] As an added precaution the vaccine was inactivated with 0·1% formalin. In 35 out of 46 people vaccinated an antibody response was induced. No adverse reactions occurred. Although these results are encouraging, their preliminary nature must be emphasised. In particular, the difficulty of ensuring complete inactivation of the virus and the possibility that host components may be present in the vaccine inducing harmful immunological reactions have been pointed out. Nevertheless, the way is clear for further work in this important area and, far from being a pariah, the healthy HBsAg carrier, through being the source of a hepatitis B vaccine, may help to eradicate one of the most serious infectious diseases remaining in the world.

REFERENCES

[1] Nielson, J O, *et al*, *New England Journal of Medicine*, 1971, **285**, 1157.
[2] Reed, W D, *et al*, *Lancet*, 1973, **2**, 690.
[3] Woolf, I L, Symposium on the Carrier State, Birmingham, 1974, British Society of Gastroenterology.
[4] Magnius, L O, and Espmark, J A, *Journal of Immunology*, 1972, **109**, 1017.
[5] Iwarson, S, *et al*, *British Medical Journal*, 1973, **1**, 84.
[6] Alter, H J, *et al*, *New England Journal of Medicine*, 1975, **292**, 455.
[7] Maupas, P, *et al*, *Lancet*, 1976, **1**, 1367.

Constipation and laxative abuse

KIKO RUTTER, DOUGLAS MAXWELL

Normal defecation is characterised by the easy, regular, and complete passage of formed motions. The elimination of dietary waste is a fundamental physiological process, but the range of normal bowel pattern is wide, as individual bowel habit is determined by cultural, social, and psychological factors. Surveys have shown that most apparently healthy people have a bowel action between three times a day and three times a week.[1] Medical opinion has now swung away from its earlier rigid insistence on the need for a regular bowel action, and there is no evidence that infrequent bowel motions cause autointoxication or result in various common symptoms such as headache and lassitude. Nevertheless, this widespread misconception, fostered by popular myth and assiduous advertising, dies hard among the public. In a survey of Londoners[2] over 30% were found to be self-medicating with laxatives, and in both Britain and the United States vast sums are spent yearly on prescribed and over-the-counter cathartics. For most people this drug habit is quite unnecessary. Although a harmless waste of money in most cases, laxative abuse by a few patients constitutes an appreciable health hazard.

PHYSIOLOGY OF DEFECATION

Rational treatment of the various forms of constipation depends on understanding normal and disordered colonic physiology. Two aspects are briefly considered here.

Colonic motility and transport—After absorption of nutrients in the small intestine the residue is presented to the colon, where further absorption of water and electrolytes takes place. Waste material is moved towards the rectum by several types of motor activity, including tonic contraction, segmentation, and transport (peristalsis or less commonly mass movement). Much recent understanding of colonic activity has been derived from measuring intraluminal pressures. From such studies has come the concept of "paradoxical motility." High intraluminal pressures (as may occur in diverticular disease and the irritable colon syndrome) may indicate slow or absent transport, as high pressures are generated by decreased volume together with an obstruction to the outlet. Conversely, rapid transport occurs in the absence of outlet obstruction, so that any pressure gradient will result in rapid movement of contents. Thus constipation, which is popularly thought to result from a lax, atonic colon, may also be associated with a hypersegmenting, high-pressure bowel. (Similarly, diarrhoea may occur in patients with a tube-like, low-pressure colon.) The practical implication of these findings is that while antispasmodics may be beneficial in constipation associated with high intraluminal pressure the use of stimulant laxatives in this form of colonic dysmotility is irrational.

Mechanism of defecation—Continence is maintained by the anal sphincters and the flap-valve mechanism of the anorectal angle. As the rectum fills and becomes distended the desire to defecate occurs and the reflex is started. The sphincters and puborectalis relax, abdominal and chest wall muscles contract, intra-abdominal pressure increases, and the rectum is evacuated. Defecation may be voluntarily inhibited, and an important factor in the development of constipation is the failure to answer the call to stool. If this is persistently ignored the sensory stimuli evoked by rectal distension eventually are suppressed and reflex defecation is inhibited.

CONSTIPATION

True constipation may be defined as a decrease in the frequency of bowel movements accompanied by the difficult passage of excessively hard stools. Defecation is prolonged and may be accompanied by local anorectal pain and a sense of incomplete evacuation.[3] Indeed, severe constipation, especially in the elderly, may result in impaction of rock-like faeces in the rectum and be associated with spurious diarrhoea.

Most people who claim to be "constipated" probably do not satisfy any reasonable definition of this disorder. When true constipation exists most patients belong to the category of simple or primary constipation (appendix I). They often give a long history and have no underlying colonic or systemic disease. The problem may be regarded as another disorder of affluent life-style, which results from a combination of inadequate bulk in the diet, insufficient exercise, and persistent failure to answer the call to stool.

Occasionally constipation is due to some disorder of colonic motility. Although the underlying motor disturbances are poorly understood, some forms are considered to result from hypomotility—for example, constipation in pregnancy and idiopathic slow-transit constipation (diagnosed by the slow transit of radio-opaque markers). A different form of colonic dysmotility probably accounts for constipation in the irritable bowel syndrome and diverticular disease. Here excessive disorderly motor activity (paradoxical motility) results in areas of high pressure and hypersegmentation and accounts for these patients associating abdominal pain with constipation.

Constipation is also recognised as a complication of various organic diseases (both local and systemic) and often accompanies certain psychiatric disorders. Finally, an iatrogenic explanation for constipation should always be considered and a careful drug history taken.

MEDICATION

The terms aperient, cathartic, evacuant, laxative, and purgative are used synonymously to describe agents that promote evacuation of the bowel. An extraordinary range of drugs is available for constipation: the current edition of the *British National Formulary* lists 14 approved preparations, while the *Monthly Index of Medical Specialities* describes 45 proprietary preparations. In the United States over 700 different over-the-counter laxative preparations are available.

Although many laxatives may have more than a single mode of action, agents used in treating constipation may be conveniently (if arbitrarily) classified in five main categories—namely, bulk producers, stool softeners, lubricants, osmotic agents, and chemical stimulants (appendix II). In addition to these agents, compounds given per rectum include fluid and lubricant enemas and suppositories containing stool softeners and irritants.

Bulk producers

Western diet has undergone profound changes in the past century, principally caused by increased consumption of sugar, fat, and processed foods and by a reduction in unabsorbed dietary fibre (roughage). Although it is difficult to consider any one of these items in isolation, epidemiological studies suggest that the low fibre content in refined foods of industrialised countries may be an important contributory factor in various bowel disorders, including appendicitis, diverticular disease, irritable bowel syndrome, and even colonic cancer. These speculations are unproved, but there is little doubt that fibre affects bowel habit and is often an effective remedy for constipation.[4] Recent studies, for example, have shown that the daily addition of 10 g unprocessed millers' wheat bran and the substitution of wholemeal bread for white bread increased daily faecal weight, softened the stools, and decreased mean intestinal transit time by almost 30% in a group of schoolboys.[5]

The precise mechanism of action of a high-fibre diet on intestinal physiology is unknown. Undoubtedly fibre-containing foodstuffs are hydrophilic, retain water in the bowel, and tend to soften the faeces. Other properties, however, such as binding of the bile salts and increasing faecal output of volatile fatty acids, may contribute to the cathartic effect.[4]

Dietary fibre is an ideal and natural source of increased bulk, and the most convenient source of crude fibre is a breakfast cereal containing bran. For patients who have difficulty in getting enough fibre-containing foodstuffs, however, several processed preparations are available (appendix II). All hydrophilic bulk laxatives should be taken with plenty of fluid to prevent obstructing boluses forming, and the dose adjusted until the required effect is obtained. They should not be prescribed for any patient with stenosing or obstructing intestinal lesions but are otherwise safe, and as the most physiological form of laxative they are suitable for long-term use should this be necessary.

Stool softeners

Stool softeners are surface-active agents on account of their detergent properties. They allow water to penetrate the faecal masses, causing stool softening, and also increase permeability of gut mucosa. They are commonly used with stimulant laxatives—for example, bisacodyl-dioctyl (Dulcodos) and danthron-poloxalkol (Dorbanex)—and are undoubtedly effective. A theoretical objection to these drugs, however, concerns their possible deleterious effect on intestinal absorption. As long-term ingestion of agents that affect surface tension may be harmful, the use of stool softeners should be restricted to patients with hard faecal masses, particularly when associated with painful anorectal disease.[3]

Lubricants

The continuous use of lubricants such as liquid paraffin or mineral oils no longer has any place in treating constipation. In effective dosage anal seepage is an unpleasant side effect and, particularly in elderly and debilitated patients, there is a real risk of aspiration and lipid pneumonia. Interference with absorption of fat-soluble vitamins has been reported, and there appears to be a slightly increased risk of developing gastrointestinal malignancy.[3]

Osmotic agents

Osmotic agents are unabsorbed solutes that retain water in the small bowel and increase the flow of fluid into the colon. In effective doses these agents may result in urgency and fluidity of stools.

Apart from the unpleasant effect of a liquid purge, excessive absorption of sodium or magnesium ions may pose a threat, particularly to patients with cardiac or renal failure. Although useful for acute evacuation of the bowel, they do not encourage a return to normal function (unlike the bulk purgatives) and have no place in the long-term management of constipation. Their routine use should be confined to evacuation of the bowel for endoscopic procedures and in the prophylaxis of hepatic coma.

Lactulose is a synthetic disaccharide (galactose+fructose). As there is no corresponding disaccharidase in the small bowel to hydrolyse this sugar it reaches the colon virtually unchanged. There it is broken down by bacteria to non-absorbable organic anions with a resultant osmotic catharsis (simulating the effect of lactose in people with lactase deficiency). Recent trials have established that lactulose is an effective although expensive laxative, and it is claimed to be more acceptable than conventional osmotic purgatives. The role of this relatively new agent, however, is not yet established. It may have a place in treating elderly or debilitated patients who do not respond satisfactorily to stimulant laxatives.

Chemical stimulants

Various compounds belong to the chemical stimulant group, some having been known since antiquity. Although the precise mode of action of these drugs is not clear, they all stimulate peristalsis by direct contact with colonic mucosa. In addition to stimulating gut motility these chemicals interfere with normal salt and water absorption.[3] They should be prescribed when the colon contains an adequate amount of bulk. The effect of most of these drugs is delayed for six to nine hours, so they should be taken in the late evening.

Stimulant laxatives are undoubtedly effective but should be used with caution, as they all produce undesirable and occasionally dangerous side effects. Taken regularly they may be habit-forming and can produce electrolyte disturbances, histological changes (melanosis coli), and even structural damage with toxic degeneration of myenteric plexuses, and eventually severe and permanent interference with colonic motility.[6]

Some of the drugs in this category are best avoided completely. Oxyphenisatin is now known to cause both acute and chronic hepatitis (the latter closely resembling chronic active liver disease) and has now been withdrawn from use in Britain. Castor oil, which has a rapid action, stimulates both small-bowel and large-bowel peristalisis, causing painful contractions, and is thus not suitable for routine use. Phenolphthalein should be avoided because of its propensity to cause fixed drug eruptions but is still widely available in many proprietary mixtures. The effectiveness of bile salts in treating constipation has recently been confirmed in a trial of cholic acid. Their long-term effects are unknown, however, and until they have been shown to be safe and to have definite advantages over established drugs they are best avoided. Of the stimulant laxatives only senna derivatives and bisacodyl can be recommended for general use, and then ideally only for short periods.

MANAGEMENT OF CONSTIPATION

When true constipation does exist an attempt must be made to achieve a specific diagnosis. Patients should be questioned about their general health, frequency and character of bowel motion, associated abdominal pain, nature of diet, occupation, and any drug treatment. Constipation associated with weight loss, abdominal pain, or fresh rectal bleeding, particularly in the elderly, should alert the doctor to possible serious organic disease. Ideally, all patients should have an abdominal and rectal examination to exclude any local rectal or anal lesion. If the rectum is loaded with faeces it is likely that reflex defecatory mechanisms have become dulled and that bowel re-education rather than medication will be required.

Simple measures

In practice, constipation is usually primary or caused by some disorder of colonic motility (appendix I). When an organic cause has been excluded the patient should be reassured that although a daily bowel movement may be desirable it is by no means essential and that a less frequent bowel motion may be quite normal for many people.

Patients with simple constipation need advice about the importance of re-establishing a satisfactory bowel habit without the need for regular laxatives. The call to stool should never be ignored, however inconvenient this may be, and time should be allowed for unhurried defecation. Patients should be advised to take more exercise and to increase their intake of fluid and unabsorbed dietary fibre—for example, with wholemeal bread, bran, or bran-based cereals.

Loaded colon

Before these simple adjustments to life-style are effective in re-establishing a satisfactory bowel habit it may be necessary to empty a loaded or impacted rectum, especially in elderly or debilitated patients. Various therapeutic measures are useful. These usually include initial treatment with a stool softener or other laxative, followed by suppositories (glycerin, bisacodyl) or by evacuant enemas (arachis oil retention enema, phosphates enema). In addition, digital evacuation may be needed. Tap water or soapy water enemas should no longer be used because of the risk of water intoxication.

Regular laxative treatment

Patients with primary constipation should not need regular laxatives. If the simple measures outlined above are unsuccessful, however, some form of bulk laxative may be needed, at least temporarily. Stimulant cathartics should be avoided both in these patients and in those with the irritable bowel syndrome. Nevertheless, they may be useful when there is diminished colonic motor response to increased luminal bulk, as occurs in elderly or debilitated patients, or in those with idiopathic slow-transit constipation. Standardised senna (Senokot) is probably the most acceptable stimulant preparation. Osmotic and lubricant laxatives are not recommended for regular use.

In a brief review such as this only general guidelines are presented.

A more detailed discussion, with particular reference to specialties such as paediatrics and obstetrics, is available.[3]

LAXATIVE ABUSE

The long-term use of laxatives ultimately leads to increasing constipation and the resort to even stronger purges. Eventually continuing catharsis itself becomes a health hazard. The syndrome of laxative abuse is now well documented, and two groups of patients at risk have been recognised.[6]

The first group includes patients with a long history of chronic constipation and increasing dependence on laxatives. With time the response to drugs is diminished, possibly as a result of damage to intrinsic nerve plexuses in the gut. Laxatives are then taken in increasing doses and variety. Ultimately the colon, especially on the right side, may become atonic and dilated—the so-called cathartic colon. These patients are often helped by withdrawing irritant drugs and substituting a high-residue diet and osmotic laxatives. If the colon has been irreversibly damaged, however, colectomy and ileorectal anastomosis may be needed.

A second group, usually women, take laxatives inappropriately and may go to great lengths to conceal the habit. Most of these women have some form of personality disorder, and with their recurrent vomiting, pathological desire to lose weight, and illicit use of diuretics closely resemble patients with anorexia nervosa. They usually present with unexplained vague ill health and serious electrolyte imbalance. Continued fluid and electrolyte depletion may result in thirst, apathy, weakness, cramps, polyuria, impaired renal function, and secondary hyperaldosteronism. Steatorrhoea, protein-losing enteropathy, and osteomalacia have all been described. Although melanosis coli may be a valuable diagnostic clue on rectal biopsy, the radiological features of cathartic colon are seldom seen. Diagnosis may be difficult and treatment of the psychological disorder often unsatisfactory. Nevertheless, if patients can be persuaded to discontinue self-medication bowel habit can rapidly return to normal.

REFERENCES

1. Connell, A M, *et al*, *British Medical Journal*, 1965, **2,** 1095.
2. Lader, S. *Practitioner*, 1965, **194,** 132.
3. Avery Jones, F, and Godding, E W, (editors), in *Management of Constipation*. London, Blackwell Scientific, 1972.
4. Cummings, J H, *Gut*, 1973, **14,** 69.
5. Payler, D K, *et al*, *Gut*, 1975, **16,** 209.
6. Cummings, J H, *Gut*, 1974, **15,** 758.
7. Hinton, J M, in *Management of Constipation*, ed F Avery Jones and E W Godding. London, Blackwell Scientific, 1972.

Constipation and laxative abuse

APPENDIX I—*Classification of constipation**

Primary (simple) constipation
- Ignoring call to stool
- Inadequate bulk in diet
- Lack of exercise
- Unfavourable working/living/lavatory facilities

Secondary to motility disorder
- Dysmotility: irritable bowel syndrome, diverticular disease
- Hypomotility: idiopathic slow transit, idiopathic megabowel, pregnancy, and elderly

Secondary to psychiatric disorder
- Depression and other chronic psychoses
- Anorexia nervosa
- Illicit laxative abuse

Secondary to known organic disease
- Colonic/rectal disease: obstructing lesions, Hirschsprung's disease, Chagas's disease
- Painful anal disease: fissure/abscess
- Endocrine/metabolic: dehydration, hypothyroidism, hypercalcaemia, lead poisoning, acute porphyria
- Neurological disease: paraplegia, multiple sclerosis

Iatrogenic disease
- Postoperative: pain, immobilisation, fluid depletion, bed-pan use
- Drug-induced: aluminium-containing antacids, codeine, hypotensives, anticholinergics, etc

* Modified from data given by Hinton.[7]

APPENDIX II—*Classification of laxatives*

Bulk producers
- Dietary fibre (bran, bran-based cereals, wholemeal bread)
- Mucilaginous polysaccharides from seeds and gums (Metamucil, Isogel, Normacol)
- Methylcellulose (Celevac)

Stool softeners
- Synthetic surface-active agents (dioctyl sodium sulphosuccinate (Dioctyl), poloxalkols)

Lubricants
- Liquid paraffin
- Mineral oil-hydrocarbon mixtures (Agarol, Petrolagar)

Osmotic agents

- Sodium, potassium, and magnesium salts (magnesium sulphate, Epsom salts; magnesium hydroxide, Milk of Magnesia; sodium potassium tartrate, Rochelle salt)
- Lactulose (Duphalac, Gatinar)

Chemical stimulants

- Anthracene compounds (senna, Senokot; danthron, Dorbanex; cascara)
- Polyphenolic compounds (bisacodyl, Dulcodos, Dulcolax; phenolphthalein—for example, Agarol, Alophen, Veracolate; oxyphenisatin, Bydolax, Cirotyl, Contax—all now withdrawn in UK)
- Castor oil
- Bile salts (cholic acid; dehydrocholic acid, Dehydrocholin; mixtures: Taxol, Veracolate)

Treatment of diarrhoea

DION R BELL

The treatment of diarrhoea includes three major elements: symptomatic, supportive, and specific. Specific treatment will, of course, depend on an accurate aetiological diagnosis, and it is only realistic to accept the fact that in most brief episodes of diarrhoea the cause is not found. For this reason, symptomatic and supportive treatment are especially important—all the more because most acute episodes of diarrhoea are self-limiting, and the patient will have recovered before rational specific treatment based on a correct diagnosis can be started.

SYMPTOMATIC TREATMENT

Symptomatic treatment aims to stop the diarrhoea, or at least reduce its severity. The traditional remedies are kaolin mixture and chalk mixture. Although they are often said to absorb "toxins" from the gut, there is little evidence to support this. The morphine present in the chalk and opium mixture and kaolin and morphine mixture acts only via the bloodstream after being absorbed from the bowel, and not by a local effect on the gut wall. As the kaolin and morphine mixture contains only 0·7 mg of morphine in 10 ml, the amount of morphine in normal doses is therapeutically insignificant. Chalk and opium mixture contains 5 mg of morphine in 10 ml, and a small but useful pharmacological effect might result from the opium absorbed.

Codeine is of little use in controlling acute diarrhoea, but it has a place in the symptomatic treatment of chronic diarrhoea, when up to 60 mg four-hourly may be used for adults.

Morphine by injection produces good symptomatic relief in acute diarrhoea associated with pain, but its use should be confined to patients with severe symptoms, such as in severe bacillary dysentery. It is usually unnecessary to give more than two or three doses. Because of its habituating potential it has no part to play in treating chronic diarrhoea.

Diphenoxylate and atropine (Lomotil) is nowadays popular, especially in keeping the patient with mild diarrhoea of short duration ambulant. The dose is two to three tablets (each contains 2·5 mg diphenoxylate) immediately, then one to two tablets six-hourly. The drug depresses the central nervous system and should not be given at the same time as other sedatives, and it can potentiate the effects of alcohol dramatically. Because of its depressant effects its use in children is no longer recommended by most paediatricians. It should not be given for more than five days and has no place in prophylaxis. The side effects of diphenoxylate, mainly drowsiness, dizziness, depression, and nausea can be troublesome. The drug is related to morphine and pethidine, so long-term administration may cause habituation. Over-dosage may cause coma and respiratory depression, reversible by nalorphine, and, preferable because of its own freedom from depressive effects, naloxone. A dose of only six tablets in a 2-year-old child led to coma and respiratory and cardiac arrest, so patients given the drug must be told of the importance of keeping it away from children. Diphenoxylate is contra-indicated if liver disease is present.

Hydrophilic substances given by mouth will absorb water from a liquid stool and themselves swell and add body to the faeces. Examples of such substances are a powder containing psyllium hydrophilic mucilloid and dextrose (Metamucil), methylcellulose granules, ispaghula husk (Isogel), and various preparations of sterculia. Their main use is the symptomatic management of chronic diarrhoea and in patients with ileostomies, and they are not usually helpful in treating acute diarrhoea.

SUPPORTIVE TREATMENT

Supportive treatment is directed towards controlling the secondary ill effects produced by the diarrhoea itself, primarily loss of water and electrolytes. All patients with diarrhoea lose excess water and electrolytes, and while the drinking of water should be encouraged—and will replace water loss adequately provided vomiting is not present—water alone is not enough except in mild cases. For mild to moderate acute diarrhoea, half physiological saline (or its equivalent) is an adequate replacement fluid. This strength of brine, about 0·45%, is not strong enough to cause nausea, and if renal function is normal it is sufficiently concentrated to keep pace with salt loss. It may be given by diluting physiological saline with an equal volume of water, and need not be sterile when given by mouth. This is an extravagant way of preparing the solution, however, and it is much more economical to advise the patient to drink water with one level medicinal teaspoon (5 g) of table salt dissolved in 1·25 l (two pints) of water. This slightly salty beverage may be made much more palatable by adding concentrated fruit cordial. The flavour combination of salt and lime juice is so pleasant that it is widely drunk from choice in SE Asia. The use of a fruit juice as an additive has the further advantage that fruit juices contain useful amounts of potassium—cheap fruit squashes often do not: a typical example analysed contained only 1·7 mmol of potassium/litre of diluted drink.

A saline solution suitable for oral fluid and salt replacement may also be made acceptable by using meat extract such as Bovril to make a bouillon. The usual strength—half a teaspoonful to the cup—again approximates to half physiological saline. ("Strong" Bovril, made by adding a large overfilled domestic teaspoon to a 200 ml cup is hypertonic and contains 188 mmol of sodium and 24 mmol of potassium/litre.)

Oral rehydration in acute diarrhoea may be made more effective by adding dextrose to the oral fluid. This is related to the effect of dextrose on electrolyte transport across the mucosa of the small intestine, one molecule of dextrose taking with it one sodium ion, both components being absorbed very rapidly. This fact is important in treating cholera and other conditions causing severe diarrhoea, and for this reason one half physiological saline in dextrose (sodium chloride 0·45% and dextrose 2·5%) is often preferred to saline alone. Sucrose normally achieves the same effects because it is rapidly hydrolysed into dextrose and fructose in the upper intestine, but in disease states the hydrolytic enzymes may be lacking, in which case sucrose will actually aggravate diarrhoea.

Rules governing the quantities of fluid needed for oral fluid and electrolyte replacement are difficult to define precisely, but as it is virtually impossible to produce overloading by the oral route, the emphasis should be on a high intake in acute diarrhoea. If oral fluid replacement of three litres a day in an adult in Britain cannot keep pace with fluid loss, and signs of dehydration develop, then admission to hospital for parenteral fluid replacement will be necessary.

Ideally, fluids intended for oral rehydration should have a similar ionic composition to the fluid lost from the gut. This varies to some extent with the site of fluid loss but always contains bicarbonate and potassium in addition to sodium and chloride. Bicarbonate can be added to "home made" solutions in the form of baking soda—sodium bicarbonate. But in domestic practice in Britain the added complication is probably not worthwhile in adults, especially as the possibility of dangerous confusion with sodium carbonate (washing soda) exists.

There are several proprietary oral rehydration fluids, but there is only one *British National Formulary* preparation—sodium chloride and dextrose compound powder. This contains, when a 22 g unit of powder is made up to 500 ml of solution, sodium 35 mmol/l, potassium 20 mmol/l, chloride 37 mmol/l, bicarbonate 18 mmol/l, and dextrose 200 mmol/l. It is quite satisfactory for oral rehydration in adults with mild or moderate dehydration, but has no noticeable advantage over the more homely remedies in the typical mild case that the doctor decides to treat at home. The powder is not always readily available, and its main usefulness is in treating infants and small children.

In chronic diarrhoea the problems of supportive treatment become more complex. This is because deficits that may be tolerated for short periods become clinically important if prolonged. These include deficits of potassium, magnesium, and bicarbonate ions in simple diarrhoea, and deficits of specific nutriments when malabsorption is present. The most important of these are iron, folate, vitamin D, and vitamin B_{12}. A regimen that includes systematic replacement of these substances has to be devised when managing chronic diarrhoea, and when malabsorption is the problem replacement usually has to be parenteral.

SPECIFIC TREATMENT

Treatment of the cause of diarrhoea can be rational only if the cause is identified. There is seldom justification for giving "specific" treatment if the cause is only conjectural, but there are exceptions. I shall mention these under the broad diagnostic categories that follow.

Acute infective diarrhoea

Although acute infective diarrhoea is not aetiologically homogenous, it is usually clinically recognisable. And it is at the stage of initial clinical "categorisation"—rather than full diagnosis—that treatment has to start. What usually puts the patient in this broad category is the presence of one or more of the following features: sudden onset, fever, malaise, vomiting, and the simultaneous occurrence of other cases sharing the same exposure. One decision of prime importance is whether or not to admit the patient to hospital.

Hospital admission should be arranged for any patient whose diarrhoea is of such severity that it seems likely that deyhdration will not be controlled by oral rehydration. The decision whether or not to admit will often be deferred until 24 hours or longer spent in observing the patient's progress. The relatives should be warned of the signs of deterioration in the patient's condition, instructed carefully in the oral rehydration procedure, and given a telephone number to ring in case of anxiety. Among the danger signs, persistent vomiting, continuing fever, and abdominal pain are the main indications for a request for another visit. None of them should be ignored.

Symptoms—It is safe to give chalk or kaolin mixture in such cases. It is probably best not to give the mixtures containing opium, and if symptoms are so severe that parenteral morphine is considered advisable, the patient should be in hospital. I believe diphenoxylate should be reserved for diarrhoea that is a social embarrassment only—such as on holiday or when attending a conference—and that it should not be given when symptoms are severe enough to put the patient to bed.

Supportive treatment—If the patient is not vomiting oral fluid and electrolyte replacement is usually sufficient. Half physiological saline is usually adequate in adults; in children, half-strength Darrow's solution is often preferred, because it contains appreciable amounts of potassium (18 mmol/l) and also lactate (25 mmol/l), which help to combat metabolic acidosis; sodium chloride and dextrose compound powder, in solution, is an alternative. If the patient feels like food this should be given. There is no need to starve a patient just because he has diarrhoea, and an adequate intake of calories will help to reduce the period of convalescence. Milk, for reasons I shall mention later, is best withdrawn from the diet temporarily.

Specific treatment—As aetiological diagnosis is seldom confirmed in the acute stages, specific treatment is based on shrewd clinical diagnosis rather than on scientific fact. But the subject is difficult, and it is often better to do nothing than to embark on empirical treatment. These are the reasons why: if the cause of the diarrhoea is salmonella food poisoning, then specific treatment—even with an antibiotic to which the organism is fully sensitive—will not shorten the duration of the diarrhoea—and worse, giving an antibiotic helps to perpetuate the carrier state. In classic salmonella food poisoning there is an explosive outbreak of diarrhoea in people exposed to a common risk, and typically the diarrhoea is preceded by fever in at least some of them. Spontaneous recovery—aided by supportive treatment—is the rule.

Some patients infected with salmonella food poisoning organisms are unable to confine the infection to the gut but suffer from a bacteraemia. This produces invasive salmonellosis, a disease similar to typhoid fever, and the systemic nature of the infection makes effective specific antibiotic treatment mandatory. The main signs of invasive disease are prolonged fever (more than 24 hours), a state of "toxic" prostration, the appearance of red macular spots, enlargement of the spleen, and meningism. Patients who develop this syndrome should be admitted to an infectious diseases unit, where they will receive an appropriate antibiotic and carefully monitored supportive treatment.

When diarrhoea of sudden onset is bloody and accompanied by fever, the most likely cause is bacillary dysentery. This suggests a shigella infection more aggressive than the *Shigella sonnei* most commonly originating in Britain. This picture is most often seen in people recently arrived from abroad—or those in contact with such people. *Shi flexneri* and *Shi dysenteriae* are the main pathogens implicated, and the infections are highly transmissible.

Again, admission of such patients to an infectious diseases unit is advisable. Those with more severe disease will need parenteral fluid replacement, and an appropriate antibiotic chosen on the basis of experience will help to shorten the illness. Shigellae are commonly resistant to sulphonamides, and ampicillin, co-trimoxazole, and nalidixic acid are the agents most likely to be effective.

The acute onset of ulcerative colitis may present in exactly the same way as bacillary dysentery; the natural history of the illness usually reveals its nature.

Diarrhoea after an acute episode

After the acute symptoms of an attack of infective diarrhoea have subsided, it is quite common to have persisting diarrhoea of lesser severity. Usually this will settle spontaneously in two or three weeks, during which time the patient may be treated symptomatically. Sometimes it does not, and the diarrhoea may then be the result of a temporary, disaccharidase deficiency in the mucosa of the small intestine. The commonest deficiency is of lactase, and the diarrhoea will then settle if lactose is removed from the diet. The main source of lactose is milk itself, as lactose has been converted into lactic acid in yoghurt and most cheeses. It is usually best to avoid milk for four weeks, then gradually introduce it in increasing amounts. Many tablets and capsules contain lactose as an excipient, often more than 0·5 g, so these should be avoided too.

Occasionally ulcerative colitis seems to be started by an attack of acute infective diarrhoea. The passage of mucus and blood indicate that this is likely and that further investigations are needed.

Diarrhoea with blood

Apart from bacillary dysentery, when fever usually precedes or accompanies the onset of diarrhoea, there are several causes of bloody diarrhoea in an afebrile patient. These include amoebic dysentery, carcinoma of the large bowel, ulcerative colitis, and even simple diarrhoea in a patient with piles. It is vital to establish the cause of the symptoms in all patients presenting in this way, and empirical treatment has no place in managing this syndrome. In aged patients faecal impaction with a stercoral ulcer may cause this picture, which can then be relieved by enemas or manual evacuation.

Amoebic dysentery

The diagnosis of amoebic dysentery has to be made by finding the amoebae, and the possibility should be considered in every patient before diagnosing ulcerative colitis, especially if the patient has lived in the tropics at any time. Rapid clinical response is produced by metronidazole 800 mg three times daily for five days, but complete eradication of the infection cannot be guaranteed with metronidazole alone, so tetracycline 0·5 g four times daily for two weeks or entamide furoate (Furamide) 0·5 g three times daily for two weeks should be given as well. In severe attacks, the addition of two or three daily intramuscular injections of 65 mg emetine hydrochloride or 100 mg dehydroemetine will accelerate clinical recovery.

Ulcerative colitis and carcinoma

At present the treatment of carcinoma must be surgical. Fortunately, only a few patients with ulcerative colitis fail to respond to medical measures, and sulphasalazine (Salazopyrin) is the most useful drug for maintenance treatment. A dose of 2 g daily will often maintain a patient in remission for years, or even for life. It is important to remember that if the inflammatory process in ulcerative colitis is not controlled then carcinoma commonly supervenes. The advantages of elective colectomy in ulcerative colitis uncontrolled by drugs are mainly two: the removal of the danger of colonic neoplasia and the greatly reduced mortality when compared with that of emergency colectomy. But if neoplastic risk is to be eliminated total colectomy must be carried out and the patient condemned to a permanent ileostomy. Decisions of such gravity must be left to experts, with the patient's informed participation. Other patients with ileostomies can play a vital part in showing that ileostomy is compatible with a full and happy life. Exactly the same approach is used when permanent colostomy after surgery for large bowel carcinoma is planned.

Recurrent diarrhoea

Recurrent diarrhoea with blood is a common feature of carcinoma, ulcerative colitis, and amoebiasis. These I have already mentioned. Recurrent diarrhoea without blood is most commonly due to the irritable bowel syndrome, but sometimes to Crohn's disease. Although the aetiology of the irritable bowel syndrome—in which diarrhoea and and constipation often alternate, and abdominal pain is common—is not known, many patients obtain relief from increasing their dietary intake of bulk-forming agents such as wheat bran. Small doses of a tranquilliser such as diazepam also often help, and many patients will volunteer the information that nervous stress aggravates their symptoms. For these patients firm reassurance on the absence of serious organic disease may be as important as medication.

Travellers' diarrhoea

Travellers' diarrhoea is a term used to describe the diarrhoea so commonly experienced by travellers abroad. It includes all the obvious causes of infective diarrhoea such as salmonella and shigella infections, but is probably most commonly caused by enterotoxin-producing strains of *Escherichia coli.* Occasionally a parasitic infection such as malaria or schistosomiasis can cause it. It is usually self-limiting, but a combination of triple sulphonamide and streptomycin (Streptotriad) given in the recommended doses will often shorten the attack. Travellers who have more persistent diarrhoea on return from abroad may have secondary disaccharidase deficiency, tropical sprue, or giardiasis. Giardiasis is often missed because many laboratories go straight to stool culture without preliminary stool microscopy and so miss the opportunity to see the typical cysts or trophozoites of *Giardia lamblia*. The *Giardia* infection is usually rapidly cleared up by a seven-day course of metronidazole, 400 mg three times daily. Failure is usually due to reinfection from another member of the household who is asymptomatic. It is quite often necessary to treat all members of a household simultaneously. The infection is now so common, especially in children, that it may be acquired without leaving Britain.

Tropical sprue is fairly rare in Britain, despite the many travellers returning from the tropics. Like giardiasis, it produces a fatty diarrhoea with flatus and weight loss, but it responds little, if at all, to metronidazole. It can be cured by treatment with tetracycline (250 mg four times daily) and folic acid (5 mg four times daily), which should be continued for three months. If relapse occurs treatment should be given for six consecutive months, and appropriate supportive treatment, such as iron replacement, given too.

Chronic diarrhoea

The subject of chronic diarrhoea is too large to deal with here. But all patients with chronic diarrhoea need accurate diagnosis before treatment is started, and this will usually include admission to hospital for investigation. The causes range from diabetes to tuberculosis, gluten enteropathy to aperient abuse, and I shall not list them. There is no excuse for treating chronic diarrhoea symptomatically if a proper diagnosis has not been made, as most of the causes, once identified, can be effectively dealt with.

I am grateful to Dr W H Taylor, consultant pathologist, for carrying out the analyses of Bovril and orange squash referred to.

Treatment of intestinal worms

H M GILLES

Most of the intestinal worms that affect man live unobtrustively in the gut and do little to impair the health of their host. Symptoms and signs usually appear only with heavy infections. Rapid air travel and the greater immigration into Europe from the tropics in recent years has resulted in helmintic infections, some of them long-standing and serious in their pathological effects, being increasingly encountered in Britain.

While infections with particular types of worms are sometimes patchy in distribution and vary greatly in intensity in different localities, in rural areas of the tropics many of the inhabitants harbour one or more intestinal worms. In non-endemic areas it is justifiable to treat all infections however light, while in areas where reinfection is likely to occur only heavy or moderate infections are worth treating unless simultaneous attempts are also made to improve environment hygiene. In endemic areas, therefore, the main aim of anthelmintic treatment should be to reduce the load of infection below the level of clinical significance. Complete parasitological cure is unnecessary. Nevertheless, in patients who are severely ill from other causes such as protein-calorie malnutrition, marasmus, tuberculosis, or sickle-cell anaemia worm infections, however light, should be treated even though reinfection is certain to occur.

In the past, laxatives before and after treatment were routinely given; they are now usually considered unnecessary except in the presence of constipation. Davis[1] has written an excellent monograph on drug treatment in intestinal helminthiases.

ASCARIASIS

At least four drugs are available for treating ascariasis; starvation before treatment is unnecessary.

Levamisole

Many regard levamisole as the drug of choice in ascariasis. It is given by mouth as a single dose of 2·5 mg/kg of body weight. Adverse reactions occur in about 1% of cases; they are mild, transient, and non-specific—for instance, nausea, vomiting, anorexia, abdominal discomfort, headache, or dizziness.

Piperazine derivatives

Four piperazine salts are generally available—adipate, calcium edetate, citrate, and phosphate. The most widely used preparation is piperazine citrate prepared as a flavoured syrup or as tablets, and some evidence suggests that the syrup gives slightly superior therapeutic results. Worldwide experience over more than 20 years has confirmed the excellent therapeutic and safety record of these derivatives.

An accepted and safe schedule for adults is a single oral dose of 75 mg/kg* with a maximum individual dose of 4 g. Two doses on successive days give a slightly higher cure rate.

Side effects—Nausea, vomiting, abdominal pain, and diarrhoea have occasionally been reported. Temporary ataxia has been described while large doses have occasionally caused convulsions in children. Piperazine derivatives are contraindicated in renal disease, liver disease, or epilepsy.

Pyrantel embonate

Pyrantel embonate is a relatively new synthetic anthelmintic. A single oral dose of 10 mg/kg is more effective than a single dose of piperazine.

Side effects are mild and transient and occur in about 20% of cases; they include headache, dizziness, vomiting, abdominal pains, and diarrhoea.

Mebendazole

Mebendazole is also an effective ascaricide. It is taken by mouth in a dose of 100 mg twice a day for three days.

Side effects include mild diarrhoea and abdominal pain.

ENTEROBIASIS

Although many compounds are active against *Enterobius vermicularis*, I will mention only three that combine efficacy, single-dose schedules, and mild unwanted effects. With all these drugs successful treatment can be effected only if infected members of the family are treated simultaneously. Examination for test of cure should be deferred until seven days after treatment.

Viprynium embonate

Viprynium embonate is generally regarded as the drug of choice. An acceptable and efficient dose is 5 mg base of the suspension (≡7·5 mg embonate) per kg on three occasions at 15-day intervals.

Side effects—The drug is well tolerated; nausea, vomiting, diarrhoea, and abdominal cramps occur only in a few patients. The stools may be stained and lead to red staining of underwear, a disadvantage.

* The dose is customarily expressed in terms of the hydrate equivalent; 100 mg of piperazine hydrate ≡ 125 mg citrate, 120 mg adipate, 104 mg phosphate and 214 mg calcium edetate.

Treatment of intestinal worms

Pyrantel embonate

Pyrantel embonate given as a single dose of 10 mg/kg is also effective in enterobiasis with cure rates of about 80–95%.

Mebendazole

A single oral dose of 100 mg of mebendazole repeated after one week has also given high cure rates.

TRICHURIASIS

Until recently the treatment of *Trichuris trichiura* infections has been most unsatisfactory. The only effective drug available to date is mebendazole. This is given in a dose of 100 mg by mouth twice daily for three days.

STRONGYLOIDIASIS

As with trichuriasis chemotherapy in strongyloidiasis is unsatisfactory. The most effective drug is thiabendazole with mebendazole a relatively satisfactory alternative.

Thiabendazole

Thiabendazole is at present the drug of choice. It is given by mouth at a dose of 25 mg/kg for three days (maximum dose 3 g/day). The tablets must be chewed and the drug is better tolerated if given after meals.

Side effects are fairly common. They may occur three or four hours after ingestion of the drug and include nausea, vomiting, anorexia, diarrhoea, and dizziness. Rarely, drowsiness, pruritus, xanthopsia, bradycardia, and hypotension may occur. The urine often smells of asparagus; a gelatinous olive-grey substance may be visible to the naked eye in centrifuged urine.

Mebendazole

Mebendazole is given, 100 mg twice daily, for four days.

HOOKWORM INFECTIONS

The geographical distribution of the two human hookworms, *Ancylostoma duodenale* and *Necator americanus*, used to be regarded as relatively distinct, the former being prevalent in the Far East and Mediterranean coastal regions and the latter in Central and South America and tropical Africa. During the past few decades, however, both parasites have become widely distributed throughout the tropics and subtropics, and rigid demarcations are no longer justifiable.

Several drugs are available for treating hookworm infections; their efficacy varies according to the species in question.* Repeated treatments are usually necessary except in light infections, and this generalisation is valid for all the drugs mentioned below.

For *A duodenale* infections treatment may be given with pyrantel embonate, bephenium hydroxynaphthoate, or mebendazole. For *N americanus* treatment with tetrachlorethylene, pyrantel embonate, or mebendazole is available. Drugs that have a better effect on one species usually also have some effect on the other species.

Tetrachlorethylene

Tetrachlorethylene (TCE) is possibly more effective against *N americanus* than against *A duodenale.* The dose is 0·1 ml/kg by mouth with a maximum adult dose of 5 ml. Alcohol and fats should be avoided for 24 hours before and after treatment. The drug should be taken on an empty stomach (light meal the night before), with water only for three hours after ingestion. Purging is unnecessary and may be harmful. Repeat treatment at four-day intervals is neccessary to cure heavy infections.

TCE is available as a liquid that should be stored in dark bottles in a cool environment, or as soft gelatin capsules of 0·2 ml, 1 ml, and 5 ml. Broken capsules should never be used.

Toxic effects include burning in the epigastrium, abdominal pain, nausea, and vomiting. Occasionally drowsiness, vertigo, symptoms like drunkenness, and transient syncope from hypotension have been described but are infrequent. Ideally, bed rest for four hours after treatment with TCE should be enforced, and in mass treatment patients should be advised to avoid excessive activity for the same period. Rarely TCE stimulates ascarids to migrate "en masse" and may cause intestinal obstruction, especially in children. In mixed infections of ascaris and hookworm, therefore, ascaris must be treated first with one of the drugs mentioned earlier (see ascariasis) before TCE is given.

Bephenium hydroxynaphthoate

Bephenium hydroxynaphthoate is more effective against *A duodenale* than against *N americanus.* The standard treatment is a single dose of 5 g of the salt (2·5 g base). For necator infections three daily doses of 5 g are usually needed to ensure a high cure rate. The drug in small granules is given with water on an empty stomach usually before breakfast.

Bephenium is also effective against ascarids, and this is an added advantage in mixed infections.

* Bitoscanate, given in three doses, appears to have equal effects against both species of hookworms, but this drug is not available in Britain.

Toxic effects are minimal. Nausea and vomiting may occur, and sometimes diarrhoea. Purgatives are unnecessary.

Pyrantel embonate

Pyrantel embonate is more active against *A duodenale* than against *N americanus*. In treating hookworm infections it compares favourably with bephenium and like this compound it is also active against ascaris infection. It is given as a single oral dose of 20 mg/kg.

Mebendazole

Mebendazole seems to be equally effective against *A duodenale* and *N americanus*. The standard dose is 100 mg by mouth twice a day for three days.

BROAD-SPECTRUM ANTHELMINTICS

Multiple intestinal helminth infections are common in the rural tropics. In these cases anthelmintics that are effective against more than one parasite may be useful. Even so, their activity against one species may be selectively lower than against another. Mebendazole, pyrantel embonate, and thiabendazole are good examples of broad-spectrum anthelmintics that have been used both for individual and mass treatment. When the multiple infections are generally light, the convenience, range, and economic advantages of using such compounds are well worth considering. With heavy infections, however, selective treatment for the appropriate species of helmintic infection is preferable.

INTESTINAL FLATWORMS (CESTODIASIS)

The intestinal flatworms or cestodes that give rise to disease in man are *Taenia saginata*, *Taenia solium*, *Diphyllobothrium latum*, and *Hymenolepisnana*.

TAENIASIS

One differential property of the two common parasites *T solium* and *T saginata* is that cysticercosis may follow infection with the pork tapeworm after regurgitation of the gravid proglottids into the gastroduodenum. While this is theoretically possible, few data are available on the association of cysticercosis with the taenicidal drugs mentioned below.

Niclosamide

Niclosamide is generally considered the drug of choice in treating human taeniasis, although some authorities refrain from using it in *T solium* infections.

The standard adult dose is 2 g before breakfast as two divided oral doses with a one-hour interval between the doses—that is, 1 g—1 hour interval—1 g. The tablets should be chewed thoroughly and washed down with a small draught of water. It is wise to restrict the diet to fluids only, starting from the evening before treatment.

The use of niclosamide in *T solium* infections should be attended by the following precautions: (*a*) an antiemetic drug should precede treatment, and (*b*) a saline purge should be given two hours after the taenicide to rid the bowel of all dead segments before digestion can occur.

Side effects of niclosamide are few, generally being restricted to mild gastrointestinal disturbances.

Dichlorophen

Dichlorophen has been superseded by niclosamide for treating human taeniasis. The usual recommended dose is 75 mg/kg with a maximum of 6 g for adults given either as a single dose or in three divided portions for one to three days.

Side effects are mild and include nausea, colic, diarrhoea, and occasionally vomiting. Jaundice has been rarely reported. Dichlorophen should not be used in the presence of jaundice or in any patient with overt liver disease.

FISH TAPEWORM

Niclosamide in the same dose and administered in the same way as for taeniasis is effective in treating *D latum* infections.

DWARF TAPEWORM

Niclosamide, 2 g on the first day followed by 1 g daily for the next six days, is recommended for *H nana* infections. Prolonged treatment is needed because of the presence of developing stages (onchospheres) in the jejunal villi. Retreatment a month later is recommended.

ECONOMIC CONSIDERATIONS

In many parts of the tropics economic considerations must determine the choice of drug that is given. Drugs such as tetrachlorethylene have justifiably maintained their place in both individual and mass treatment of hookworm infections for nearly 50 years on grounds of low cost, ease of administration, and tolerance.

DIAGNOSIS

The diagnosis of gastrointestinal helminthiasis depends on the demonstration of the characteristic eggs in the stool or the recovery of adult worms or segments of worms. Examination of a direct saline smear of faeces is often successful in establishing a diagnosis; alternatively, various concentration techniques are available. In some instances ancillary methods such as radiology, sigmoidoscopy, serology, or other specialised techniques are required.

Human taeniasis is commonly diagnosed through the macroscopic and microscopic identification of expelled proglottids; eggs may be present only intermittently in the stools in the presence of known infections.

REFERENCE

[1] Davis, A, *Drug Treatment in Intestinal Helminthiases*. Geneva, World Health Organisation, 1973.

Anorexia and loss of weight

CLIFFORD HAWKINS

Appetite is a pleasant sensation related to previous gustatory experiences, whereas hunger—less common in a society where eating three or four meals daily has become a social habit—is disagreeable and associated with hunger pangs sometimes caused by unrequited gastric peristalsis. Appetite bears no relation to the need of the body so the amount of food eaten by man, which depends on social and environmental factors, is usually greater than he needs. Although obese people are blamed for their unrestrained appetite, some experiments[1] suggest that they may be less influenced by their viscera than people of normal weight. Normally, eating behaviour correlates closely with gastric motility and whether the stomach is empty or full; but the feeling of satiety may be absent or take longer to develop in obese people—so there is no brake to limit the appetite. Perhaps, however, this is acquired rather than constitutional and the result of disregarding the sensation of satiety.

Appetite is rightly regarded as an index of health, hence inquiry about it is part of the routine of every case history. Yet surprisingly little is known about the physiology of appetite. Animal experiments suggest the presence of a feeding centre in the lateral hypothalamus and a satiety centre situated more medially, which, if stimulated by cold or hypoglycaemia, could activate the lateral centre. So the hypothalamus is thought to regulate eating, and clinical pointers to this are the alleged rare tumours of the pituitary gland or suprasellar region that cause the patient either to starve or to over-eat. Yet the psyche exerts great influence: for the appearance, sight, smell, colour, texture, and consistency of foods are such important external stimuli. Every dietitian knows this, and convalescent patients easily lose their appetite if served meals that are too large or look uninteresting.

The stomach itself may play only a minor part. Pavlov described the conditioned reflex sparked off by the sight of food—salivation with increased gastric tone and secretion. Patients suffering from pernicious anaemia, however, who have neither gastric acid nor pepsin eat normally unless their tongue is sore from B_{12} deficiency. Lesions of the stomach, even early cancer, do not diminish appetite. Gastritis, as seen endoscopically, is common in healthy people with normal appetite. Peptic ulcer does not cause anorexia but appetite may be depressed for fear of eating. Gastric operations such as partial gastrectomy, however, reduce appetite, probably because of an inability to eat large meals owing to the small size of the stomach. Fear inhibits motility, and sudden loss of gastric tone can be seen by the radiologist when bad news is given to someone during a barium meal; but this loss of tone may be the effect of the psyche and not the cause of anorexia, for one sees patients whose appetite is normal despite gastric hypotonia. Hypoglycaemia increases appetite, but there is no indication that hyperglycaemia depresses it—for example, the obese diabetic patient whose blood sugar is high still finds it difficult to diet.

CAUSES OF ANOREXIA

Anorexia, when it occurs alone, is usually psychogenic; but because it is an expected symptom of many conditions organic disease must be excluded. All types of fever depress appetite as do chronic inflammatory states like active rheumatoid arthritis or granulomata of the bowel such as ulcerative colitis or Crohn's disease. Abnormal metabolic states may present with anorexia. Uraemia, which also causes early morning sickness, is usually excluded by testing the urine. The apathy and anorexia of early Addison's disease may be caused by either hyponatraemia or hypercalcaemia. Hypercalcaemia can mimic neurosis by causing anorexia and depression; this occurs in sarcoidosis, hyperparathyroidism, carcinomatous deposits in the bone, excess vitamin D medication, and the milk-alkali syndrome—still occasionally seen in those who drink excess milk and take too much alkali.

Anorexia is seldom helpful in diagnosis or as a specific early symptom. It may herald acute hepatitis before jaundice appears. Mental change and loss of appetite may usher in carcinoma of the pancreas, though rarely. Patients with congestive cardiac failure are anorectic, and this is either due to gastric oedema, ascites, electrolyte changes from diuretics, or digoxin. Protein deficiency, as in kwashiorkor, causes anorexia and ultimately destroys all desire to eat. It is a late sign of carcinoma and may suggest secondary deposits in the liver.

Drugs

Anorexia, nausea, and vomiting are mentioned on almost every data sheet issued by pharmaceutical firms as possible side effects of drugs. How drugs cause this, whether they act on the stomach or brain, is virtually unknown. Nevertheless, although gastrointestinal reactions account for up to 40% of all adverse drug reactions, only a few are responsible for most. Diagnosis of drug-induced anorexia is easy if this cause is kept in mind.

Drugs that are easily overlooked are alcohol and narcotics, for addicts conceal their addiction. In hospital, digoxin causes many patients to develop anorexia due to nausea; indeed some are wrongly investigated for gastrointestinal disease or malignancy because of this. The loss of appetite is insidious and the toxic effect of digoxin may be increased by hypokalaemia, especially in the elderly. The return of appetite when the drug is stopped or the dose reduced is striking. Amphetamine and other anorectic drugs are unlikely to be overlooked, unless, for example, amphetamine is being used by an addict. Cytotoxic drugs may add to the anorexia of advanced malignant disease. Biguanides such as phenformin or metformin cause anorexia, but this may help the obese diabetic patient to reduce weight.

Nowadays more and more patients are given an ever increasing number of drugs so the possibility of drugs either alone or in combination causing anorexia must be remembered.

Dysgeusia

Disturbances of taste commonly cause anorexia, and little is known about the pathogenesis of dysgeusia. It may afflict patients when recovering from operations so that, for example, a man who normally enjoys a gin and tonic finds it too unpleasant to swallow. Sometimes, though not necessarily so, this is due to loss of large amounts of fluid and electrolytes. One study suggested that the hypogeusia that occurs after severe burns may be attributed to a disturbance of trace metals such as zinc.[2] Drugs certainly may disturb taste: chelating agents like penicillamine may cause metallic or other sensations that prevent patients eating. Sometimes the sense of taste is disturbed from psychogenic reasons or because of age. Bizarre tastes may arise in pregnancy and cause a reduced calorie intake when the woman yearns for watercress or enjoys munching coal, some even preferring the black shiny type as it tastes more crisp and nutty.

Psychogenic causes

Loss of appetite with fastidiousness about food is often part of the make-up of the neurotic patient, the extreme form being anorexia nervosa, when, without treatment, patients may starve themselves to death. Any simple worry like a forthcoming examination or marriage may cause anorexia; sometimes instant cure is possible when a patient, for example, with cancerophobia, is reassured.

Nervous dyspepsia is common; sometimes appetite may be satisfactory but feelings of fullness start after a few mouthfuls and the meal has to be stopped. Eating is further restricted because of "allergy" to various foods but this usually lies in the psyche rather than in the gastric mucosa. An indication of the nervous origin is that even the sight or smell of food causes anorexia. Depressive states often cause anorexia and weight loss. Patients may have to be investigated fully before organic disease is excluded, but diagnosis is often needlessly delayed because of the fear of missing some untreatable disease; this also inhibits a positive attitude towards the illness. Other important pointers to psychogenic disease, apart from anorexia, are unexplained tiredness, loss of interest in sex, and insomnia.

Mild cases of anorexia nervosa may be treated and cured by a sympathetic general practitioner who finds time to talk and listen. Many will need to go into hospital. This provides discipline so that the amount of food consumed can be measured and secret routes of disposal (hiding it in the locker or self-induced vomiting in the lavatory) blocked. The patient may have to be confined to bed at the start, and rewards such as increased privileges are given for gaining weight. Feeding by tube or vein is rarely done today. No specific drug is available, and management may have to go on patiently over months or years. An altered and abnormal attitude to body size may account for the morbid fear of even reaching a normal weight, apart from becoming fat. Some have suggested that the cause is a faulty setting of the regulating mechanism of appetite in the hypothalamus—the opposite to obesity; or perhaps people just develop a habit of eating too much or too little and the stomach adjusts itself accordingly. Whatever the psychological explanation, the habit of eating properly must be regained in spite of the remarkable resolution to shun food—especially anything considered fattening, such as carbohydrates. A liquid diet to begin with may help as calorie content is concealed. Later, the aim will be to give solid food with a 3000–5000 daily calorie intake.

MEASURES TO INCREASE APPETITE

The presentation of food for a sick person may easily be overlooked in hospitals, partly because of an increasing technological approach to the patient. Formerly, doctors took more interest in this and had the time to do so, and matrons, especially in small hospitals, took a personal interest in the patient's food and in supervising the cooks and service to the wards.

Appetite is depressed if food looks uninteresting (see figure), is lukewarm and tasteless, and served in too large portions. There should be close rapport between the person serving the food and the patient, so that it can be tailored to the individual need; otherwise portions are served up to frail old ladies that are more suitably for tough healthy young men recovering from a minor operation. Unfortunately the tendency is more and more for a plated meal service to be dispensed from the main kitchen and then the catering staff do not know whom they are serving. Convenience foods such as packaged frozen vegetables may be dull. The present cut-backs in spending on food has affected some patients' appetite and brought complaints. Sometimes, however, these are due to the rigid conventional eating patterns commonly seen in certain social strata: good plain food is preferred to variations liked by the gourmet—for example, rice served occasionally instead of

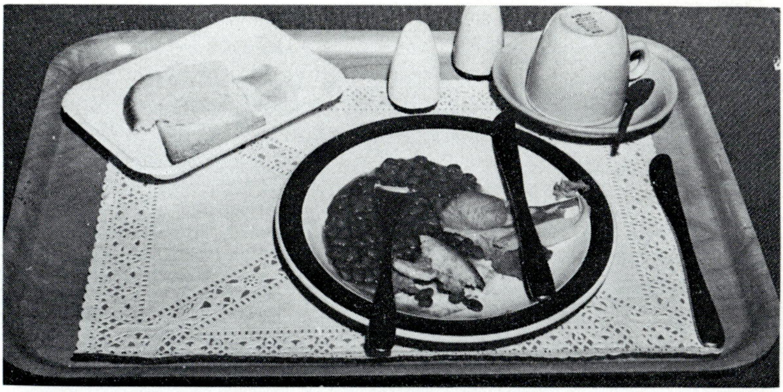

Unsuitable breakfast served inadvertently to woman with high temperature and anorexia: bacon, baked beans, cold toast without butter, and no tea or coffee.

potato was criticised. Relatives should be encouraged to bring in delicacies that the National Health Service cannot reasonably provide. Food cooked in bulk in an institution is likely to compare unfavourably with food at home. The standard of food in many hospitals, however, is remarkably good. Menus provide a choice of three or four dishes for NHS patients and the ward sister is able to supervise the type and quantity of food reaching the patient.

Fresh air, exercise, and cold are thought to stimulate appetite, and certainly many ate less during the summer heat wave. Relief of anxiety may improve appetite. This may explain the possible effect of aperitifs such as sherry; their action upon the psyche in causing relaxation is probably more important than stimulating a flow of gastric juice. Diazepam may overcome anorexia in phobic and anxiety states, and a short rest before rather than after a meal may help the tense person. Antidepressive drugs may restore appetite for the depressed.

The *British National Formulary* mentions no drugs that improve appetite—just those that depress it. Martindale's *Extra Pharmacopoeia* records prolintane hydrochloride and the antihistaminic drug cyproheptadine hydrochloride; one small drug trial suggested that the latter might be more than a placebo and increase weight by some means other than by inducing slight hypoglycaemia. *MIMS*[3] lists 11 preparations under "tonics and appetite stimulants," usually concoctions containing a mixture of vitamins and substances varying from strychnine to manganese glycerophosphates flavoured with bitters such as gentian, orange, or cherry elixir—these placebos provide a colourful link with the apothecaries of bygone days. Bitters, commonly alcoholic extracts of herbs, were used before accurate diagnosis became possible to encourage appetite and assist eructation; indeed, Hippocrates prescribed wormwood for intestinal obstruction.[4] Bitters are the basis of most tonics, and these may cost the NHS over £1m each year.[5]

Some drugs may stimulate appetite indirectly—for example, patients with anorexia nervosa have been treated by small doses of insulin in the past. Corticosteroids and corticotrophin induce a sense of well-being and so increase enjoyment of food. An elderly person suffering from polymyalgia rheumatica may improve dramatically with a small dose of prednisolone—for instance, 5 mg daily. Corticosteroids in larger doses may improve the lot of the patient dying of carcinoma and reduce temperature to normal. The Brompton Hospital mixture (listed in *BNF* under diamorphine and cocaine elixir, *BPC*) can relieve the pain and fear of advanced malignant disease so that food is again enjoyed.

LOSS OF WEIGHT

Loss of weight is usually caused by insufficient intake. This fact is sometimes difficult to uncover, and relatives may be more aware of it than the patient who hotly denies any change in eating habits; an example is bereavement. Physiological weight loss may occur at certain ages such as when a teenager leaves school to start an active job. The lay idea of good health is often that of a plump red person, a tribute to the wife's cooking. So loss of weight sometimes causes unnecessary anxiety and may even be judged by the look of the person rather than by measurement on scales.

Failure to eat may be due to causes other than anorexia, such as new dentures, painful gums, or sore tongue. Oesophageal obstruction, whether from achalasia or carcinoma, may be overlooked. Conversely, intake may be good but food is not absorbed. This happens in patients with malabsorption such as adult coeliac disease and is so common after gastric operations that patients should be warned to expect some weight loss. Obesity operations such as the 14×4 procedure when much of the small intestine is bypassed may be effective not because food passes through without absorption but because appetite is depressed owing to the operation itself.[6]

Any systemic illness is likely to cause weight reduction, partly by depressed appetite and partly from increased catabolism. Thyrotoxicosis affects catabolism only. Textbooks list numerous disorders as presenting with weight loss, especially tuberculosis and malignant disease; but this may mislead for it is not an early sign of either. Patients admitted for investigations for loss of weight with few other symptoms but a high erythrocyte sedimentation rate (Westergren) are more often found to have a connective tissue disorder than carcinoma.

Treating loss of weight alone seldom arises as it corrects itself when the underlying disease is cured or controlled. The increased catabolism with negative nitrogen balance of illnesses like granulomatous disease of the bowel or connective tissue disorders calls for adequate intake of calories with increased protein, and proprietary supplements like Casilan or Complan may be needed. Androgenic steroids, which have an anabolic effect, may be used. Wasted patients—for example, those suffering from carcinoma of the oesophagus or stomach—may need preoperative feeding[7] as this may help to counteract possible impaired wound healing and immunological defence mechanisms. When, as is often possible, this can be achieved by oral rather than intravenous feeding, the help of a dietitian in providing high calorie drinks and foods suited to the capricious appetite of these patients is invaluable.

REFERENCES

1 Schachter, S, *Science*, 1968, **161,** 751.
2 Cohen, I K, Schechter, P J, and Henkin, R I, *Journal of the American Medical Association*, 1973, **223,** 914.
3 *MIMS* (*Monthly Index of Medical Specialities*). London, Haymarket Publishing Ltd.
4 Anderson, J, *Practitioner*, 1974, **212,** 536.
5 Kinlock, J D, *Practitioner*, 1971, **206,** 44.
6 Pilkington, T R E, *et al*, *British Medical Journal*, 1976, **1,** 1504.
7 Ellis, B W, *et al*, *British Medical Journal*, 1976, **1,** 1388.

Obesity

JOHN R BENNETT, MICHAEL BADDELEY

Persuading fat people to lose weight is a task that most doctors have to undertake but few relish and none find easy. Yet it must not be shirked, for obesity affects an increasing proportion of the population and its ravages show in mortality figures for abdominal surgery, in orthopaedic clinics, in deaths from degenerative heart disease, and in bulging diabetic clinics. Actuaries are not people to be swayed by emotion, but they have demonstrated the increased mortality of fat people for many years. Now, if it is so common and so dangerous yet so obviously related to such a simple biological function as eating, why are we so poor at treating and reversing it?

ORIGIN OF OBESITY

Recent research points to the ominous likelihood that the obesity of many, perhaps most, fat adults is founded on faulty nutrition in childhood. Compounded by the vicious spiral of obesity itself leading to weight gain, the formidability of the problem becomes more evident and should encourage us to take a less casual approach to our fat patients.

Adipose tissue—The "adipose organ" is diffuse but large in volume and weighs 10–20 kg in most normal adults (10 times heavier than the liver). In obese people it may be 10 times heavier again. It is not an inert mass of fat: the triglyceride content is constantly mobilised and laid down in response to control factors that are not well understood but probably include growth hormone, noradrenaline, and other hormones.

Fat cells—Fat cells (adipocytes) are distributed throughout our bodies subcutaneously and in deeper layers, and in obesity there is an increase in their size or their number, or both. About 20% of patients fall into the first category, 10% into the second, and 70% into the last. The number of adipose cells is fairly constant in the neonate and increases steadily up to puberty. Overfeeding in neonatal life produces a more rapid increase in cell numbers, and it seems likely that the same may happen at puberty. It also seems that adipocytes do not disappear; if their number is increased, it stays large.

Two conclusions stem from these findings: firstly, that *prevention* of obesity is more important than was previously realised; and, secondly, that fat patients who were obese in childhood or adolescence will be harder to treat than those with a later onset.

Fat production—Fat is formed from triglycerides absorbed from the intestine. The amount laid down in adipocytes partly depends on the availability of carbohydrate. Carbohydrate is additionally a source of fat for deposition under the control of insulin. Thus carbohydrate has two roles in the laying down of adipose tissue, which explains why it is possible to lose weight while eating fat, provided carbohydrate sources are severely restricted.

Fat mobilisation—The adipose organ serves not only as insulation but as an energy store. Fat provides about 38 kJ (9 kcal) of energy per gram; this is consumed in about two minutes of gardening or one minute of dancing or running. That means that eight hours' running is needed to work off half a kilogram of fat; so if people are to slim it is not enough to take "a little more exercise." Nevertheless, the balance between calorie intake and energy expenditure is so fine that while exercise alone cannot be the major factor in slimming it is an important element in weight control.

FOOD INTAKE

It is a truism that the balance between food intake and energy expenditure determines the amount available for storage as fat, but many patients fail to comprehend it; some seem to believe that photosynthesis is possible in man. In our relatively affluent Western civilisation the following important factors govern food intake.

Habit—Social and family custom rather than need govern what meals we take, when we take them, and what they contain. In the industrial North it is traditional to eat high tea providing plenty of baked carbohydrates. Businessmen and politicians are increasingly exposed to large meals with alcohol. Some housewives and lorry drivers fortify themselves with multiple mugs of heavily sweetened tea. Dietary custom is the common explanation of familial obesity, though genetic factors do have an influence.

Economic—Cost comes second to habit in determining the composition of the diet. A filling and palatable meal may be prepared conveniently from carbohydrate more cheaply than from protein and vegetable, though with care the difference is small. Sometimes, therefore, obesity is a form of malnutrition, and slimming may be regarded as an expensive luxury by those on limited incomes.

Psychological—The psychological drives to eat are poorly understood, but it may easily be recognised that certain psychological and emotional states predispose to disordered eating patterns. These are unpredictable and subject to modification by circumstances. Depression may thus lead to anorexia and weight loss but equally may lead to overeating. Boredom may be relieved by eating, and food may be a form of gratification for the emotionally or sexually deprived. In all these cases altered food intake is likely to be combined with low energy expenditure.

Endocrine—Glandular trouble as the cause of obesity is a hopeful rationalisation beloved of the fat patient. Rarely is it the true reason. The occasional patient with Cushing's syndrome, hypothyroidism, gonadal failure, hypothalamic syndrome, and so forth should not long escape detection if a relatively simple history is taken and physical examination is performed.

PREVENTION

Since the number of adipocytes partly determines future body weight and their number is dependent on childhood and adolescent feeding there is much scope for preventing obesity—and this must start early. This is an educational task, but much can be done in the frequent contacts between mother and baby and doctor and nurse.

Breast-feeding carries many advantages, but the excessive weight gain of many bottle-fed babies is particularly to be deplored. In baby clinics the overweight baby is just as serious a problem as the underweight one, and compliments to the mothers of chubby babies should be kept to a minimum. The introduction of solids should be delayed until the baby is at least 3 months old.

Adolescence is the other danger period, but medical contacts are likely to be fewer. Any opportunity to diminish the excessive weight that accompanies the frequent carbohydrate ingestion at this age is to be encouraged.

THE FAT PATIENT

As in so many conditions, time devoted to the patient, particularly in the early stages, produces better results. We all have too little time, and inducing weight loss is often tedious and unappealing, so frequently we condemn ourselves (and our patients) to failure by a poor initial consultation.

Some patients will come to seek advice on slimming. They will already have tried (possibly many times) unsuccessfully, so a quick answer and a standard diet sheet will not help them.

The limited assessment suggested below serves two purposes. It will help the doctor, at least in estimating the prognosis. It will also help to impress the patient that slimming is medically important and not just another fashionable trend, such as sun-tan.

Assessment

Family history—Patients from fat families feel their obesity is inevitable. Try to establish how much is caused by family eating habits and explain the small contribution of inheritance.

Early life—Was the patient overweight as a baby, as a child, as an adolescent? If so the prognosis is less good and the task greater. It helps if patient and doctor both understand that.

Precipitating factors—Was the weight gain rapid, suggesting a specific cause—change of job, an emotional problem, reduced circumstances?

Reasons for seeking treatment

The most difficult part of treating the obese is convincing them that they need to become thinner. Time spent doing so is worth while, though constant reminders will be needed. Some patients come already motivated; they have become aware of their obesity (friends or relatives may have helped) and chiefly want advice on techniques. Even this group, though, will be helped by reminders of the virtue of weight reduction.

The others will appear because of medical problems associated with obesity—diabetes, arthritis, cardiovascular disease, reflux oesophagitis—or perhaps having been "loaded" by a life assurance company. The need for them to slim has to be explained carefully, not simply emphasising the immediate medical need but using parallel arguments such as the attractiveness of slimmer people, less difficult in finding clothes, etc.

Many patients from both groups will have made more or less serious attempts to lose weight. The reasons for failure should be explained. Poor advice on diet and failure to persist are the usual explanations.

Medical screening

A relatively elaborate programme of physical examination and special tests has the effect of emphasising the importance of the patients' obesity; some become highly motivated after experiencing one of the commercial "screening" programmes.

For the average patient in the standard busy practice a complicated programme is unjustified, but as a basis, the following are important.

Dietary history—There is no purpose in giving advice on diet if the advice is not based on a detailed knowledge of the patient's existing habits. Treatment begins here, for undesirable content in the diet can be pointed out.

Menstrual history—Major disturbances may point to an endocrine abnormality.

Brief psychiatric history—This should be taken, particularly to pick up depression, boredom, etc.

Brief physical examination—This should include blood pressure, urine test, and examination of thyroid gland, hair distribution, and testicular size (as pointers to endocrine disease).

If this screening shows any abnormalities some or all of the following procedures *may* be desirable: *x*-ray examinations of chest and skull, electrocardiography, thyroid function test, blood sugar estimation or glucose tolerance test or both, and measurement of serum lipids and cortisol levels.

TREATMENT

Mild slimming

Mild slimming is suitable for patients with a weight 20% or less above normal and with a good prognosis—that is, no family history and no early-life obesity. Put simply, it amounts to those with "middle-aged spread". They must understand that obesity will readily recur and that adjustments in the diet must be *permanent*.

For the intelligent and well-motivated quite simple advice, directed at moderate reductions in carbohydrate intake (including alcohol), is enough. Others will need a diet sheet (perhaps 4 MJ (1000 kcal)), but this must be explained verbally as well. Between-meal snacks (at home and on social occasions) are a major hazard and must be forbidden.

Exercise must be strongly recommended unless there are clear medical reasons against it. This is as useful in relieving boredom as it is in expending calories.

Increased body cooling stimulates exercise (or even shivering if it is severe enough) to maintain body temperature, and therefore increases metabolism and consequent weight loss. Fat patients should be encouraged to keep their central heating low and to wear less well-insulating clothing. Our modern tendency to accept increasingly high ambient temperatures in houses and work-places is disadvantageous to the obese.

Moderate obesity

Most moderately obese patients will have a long (often lifelong) history of obesity, many of them with a strong family history too. They will often be pessimistic about weight reduction, even resigned to its impossibility.

An important element in the philosophy with these difficult patients is to set realistic targets. If their obesity is relatively recent and not familial they may be able to get close to "ideal" weight (as in life-assurance tables), but the rest are unlikely to. Often a target mid-way between present weight and ideal weight is reasonable, provided it can be maintained. Flexibility is desirable if rapport is to continue, and even if the patient fails to reach the agreed target any weight loss is advantageous provided it is permanent.

Diet

A diet must be selected that will suit the patient's social, economic, and industrial status. There is no point in advocating expensive protein foods to the poor or advising a standard three-course lunch for a man who has to carry it to work. Neverthheless, there is much room for intelligent advice; many families are dietetically unadventurous, and the substitution of an airtight plastic container of salad for the conventional box of sandwiches might not occur to them.

There are two goals in advice on diets: one is to reduce calorie intake and induce weight loss, and the other is to change the patient's diet permanently for the better. Thus the patient who "doesn't eat a thing until teatime" (they all nibble) must be brought round to eating three standard meals. A diet sheet without explanation will be unsuccessful; so will spoken advice without a detailed written sheet for revision. By writing modifications into the diet sheet as he discusses it the doctor ensures that it fits in with the patient's needs; this also forges a closer link with the patient, who sees that the doctor cares. Initially 4 MJ (1000 kcal) is desirable, but if weight is not lost despite adhering to it 3·8 MJ (900 kcal) should be tried.

Frequent and regular assessment is vital; this need not be time-consuming. The patient should use the same machine to record his weight (not daily, because it is so variable), but the doctor should see the patient as often as progress indicates the need. Weekly visits are desirable at first, but if weight is not lost initially it never will be—and disillusionment has to be postponed as long as possible. Early weight loss will be followed by static periods, which need to be discussed. These revisits may become boring for patient and doctor alike, so different topics should be chosen for successive visits: "nibbling and its dangers," "exercise," "how to cope with eating out," "how to deal with the rest of the family," and so forth.

A useful exercise is for patients to write down in a diary exactly what they eat and drink each day, as this inhibits nibbling.

Group therapy

As in other behavioural disorders group therapy may be helpful. Doctors have rarely applied this to obesity but commercial organisations have done so successfully. Weight Watchers, *Slimming*, and other ideas may help those who can afford it and who might enjoy and benefit from social contact. Relapse is unfortunately frequent, once the patient ceases to attend. Some imitators have set up organisations that are expensive but less successful.

There is no reason why doctors should not set up their own slimming group in a group practice, with weekly meetings guided by a dietetically trained nurse.

Hypnosis and psychotherapy

Some suggestible patients feel they might benefit from hypnosis or psychotherapy. Results are generally disappointing, particularly in the long term.

Obesity

Health farms

Like any other form of temporary treatment the short-term success of expensive starvation is not well maintained.

Hormones

The use of thyroxine or sex hormones is dangerous and unhelpful.

Anorectic drugs

People do not become fat because they have abnormal hunger, and treatment based on induced anorexia is unlikely to be beneficial. Amphetamines are dangerous because of addiction (and most amphetamine-habituated patients remain fat). Their successors (fenfluramine, diethylpropion) are more acceptable but their overall value is small because of the high risk of relapse once they are stopped. The importance of a conscious and permanent change of diet cannot be overemphasised, and these drugs fail to achieve it.

Diuretics

Obesity is not caused by abnormal water retention, though fat people may have mild oedema. This will disappear as fat is lost. Diuretics give artificial weight reduction in the early stages, but when weight loss ceases after one or two weeks the disappointment is increased. Diuretics should not be used in treating obesity.

Bulk substances

Methylcellulose, as a tablet or in proprietary slimming foods, fills up the stomach and intestine by absorbing water. It makes the patient feel bloated and may relieve constipation but it does not alter his appetite. It is a harmless placebo for the patient who might be satisfied by "a pill" but is not a helpful contribution to weight loss.

Patent diets

Proprietary formula diets are best avoided. Their ability to enable the patient to lose weight if rigidly adhered to is undoubted, but they are boring, so that deviations usually occur. Moreover, they cannot be maintained permanently.

More pernicious are forms of standard food alleged to be "suitable for slimmers"; the advertising often subtly implies that the more they are eaten the thinner the eater becomes. Patent breads, drinks, and biscuits fall into this range. They are expensive and confusing to the dieter. Low-calorie fruit juices and other drinks are permissible, but many so-called "diabetic foods"—some jams, marmalades, etc—are to be avoided because of their high sorbitol content. Care must be taken if sugar substitutes are used; only those containing pure saccharin should be advised.

Reading matter

Literate patients may be helped by reading the *Which Slimming Guide* (Consumers Association, £1·75) or *Slim and Enjoy It* (Family Doctor Publications, 25p).

SEVERE OBESITY

When patients are approaching double their ideal weight or more the problem is serious, because life-threatening complications may occur. If the measures outlined above fail to achieve adequate and sustained weight reduction radical treatment may be justified.

Starvation

A nil-calorie intake will induce weight loss even in the inactive, insulated, grossly obese patient. It can be achieved only under inpatient hospital supervision to ensure careful physiological and biochemical monitoring. It is hazardous, for many patients feel ill, experience severe biochemical upsets (particularly ketosis and hypokalaemia), and some die. Provided the patients' motivation is adequate, then periods of 60 to 120 days of starvation (with an occasional low-calorie meal) will reduce their weight effectively. The danger, as with all slimming, is of relapse, particularly in the severely obese group. If weight is brought to within 25% above the ideal and subsequent outpatient supervision is maintained the prognosis is quite good.

The disadvantages, apart from the dangers listed above, are economic. The patient has to stop work and occupy an increasingly expensive hospital bed. Diversions have to be provided too. It is a form of treatment to be restricted to suitable and deserving cases only.

SURGERY

Surgical measures to aid weight reduction include panniculectomy, dieting enforced by dental splintage, gastric bypass or gastroplasty, and small-bowel bypass.

Panniculectomy

Removal of the pendulous pannicles of fat from the abdominal wall is more commonly known as "apronectomy." This and similar procedures on the breasts, arms, thighs, and legs are mainly cosmetic exercises of psychological benefit in improving the patient's own body image. Apronectomy additionally has the advantage of removing several pounds of weight, which, situated in front of the body's centre of gravity, may be a cause of backache. Otherwise, in terms of actual weight reduction, panniculectomy has little to offer.

Dental splintage

Conventional diets usually fail when provocative stresses evoke depressive mood changes resulting in a return to compulsive or episodic overeating. The depression is worsened by the consequent regain in weight or failure to achieve further reduction. Dental splintage provides a means of preventing overeating at such times of stress.

Suitable patients must have an adequate natural dentition to be able to have cap splints or interdental wires. Often preliminary dental treatment is required. The splint wires that secure the cap splints have to be removed for a few hours each month to allow jaw movements and thus prevent trismus, and the dental caps must be removed after three months for dental hygiene. A fluid diet based on milk or soups with vitamin and iron supplements and providing 3·5–4 MJ (800–1000 kcal) is continued throughout.

For those patients who last the course good weight reduction can be achieved. A controlled diet should be continued when the splints are finally removed, for otherwise lapse occurs.

About half the patients find that they cannot tolerate the fixation of their jaws or take advantage of accidental or deliberate fracture of the wires or splints to break the regimen. Thus they do not achieve the desired weight reduction and are failures.

The technique of dental splintage, though by no means inexpensive, is cheaper than therapeutic starvation, as inpatient care is avoided and minimum time is lost from work.

Gastric bypass

Polya partial gastrectomy can cause substantial weight loss by drastically reducing the gastric reservoir and by causing "dumping." These complications have been used to treat massively obese patients by 90% gastric exclusion using either transection with gastrojejunostomy or gastroplasty. The results in two series have been satisfactory but it is technically more difficult in these huge patients than small-bowel bypass and thus is less popular with surgeons.

Small-bowel bypass

Massive small-bowel resection after mesenteric vascular catastrophe is compatible with survival, albeit with a variable amount of nutritional support. A modification of this surgical emergency has been applied to the management of gross refractory obesity in the form of small-bowel bypass without resection. The duodenum and upper jejunum are retained "in circuit" for the absorption of iron, folate, and carbohydrate, and the terminal ileum for vitamin B_{12} and bile salt absorption. The absorption of fat and, to a less extent protein, is reduced by excluding much of the jejunum and most of the ileum.

Weight reduction after bypass amounts, on average, to about 36% of the original body weight. Some have lost as much as half their weight and a few very little. The latter may be caused by early resumption of voracious eating habits, slow small-bowel transit time, or insufficient bypass. Patients under 30 lose more weight than those over 50, and men lose more than women.

As this is a major operation in patients who are by definition bad risks, it might be expected that there would be a high operative or late mortality. The operative death rate is, however, surprisingly low—in the region of 1–1·5%. The late mortality, attributable largely to the metabolic effects of malabsorption, is 3–4%. There are additional risks, which all obese patients carry, of myocardial infarction and thromboembolic disease, which would occur whether or not any operation was performed.

About half the patients have some form of long-term morbidity. Diarrhoea initially is troublesome but may be adequately controlled with codeine phosphate after a few weeks or months. During this period haemorrhoids may be a nuisance. Foul flatus affects some and may be embarrassing; it is usually readily controlled with metronidazole or tetracycline in short courses repeated as necessary. Abdominal distension after meals is also not uncommon and is due to gaseous pseudo-obstruction of the colon. It too can usually be controlled with the same antibiotics.

During the first months, nausea and vomiting may be a problem needing antiemetics. It usually settles spontaneously, but when accompanied by excessive diarrhoea may require admission to hospital for two or three days of intravenous fluid and electrolyte repletion.

A puzzling complication in a few cases has been polyarthralgia, often affecting the small joints, and polymyalgia. In our experience these problems often settle with co-trimoxazole treatment but in two patients it has been necessary to reverse the operation because they proved resistant to all treatment. The restoration of normal bowel circuitary instantly eliminated the symptoms.

The main complication, and the only serious one, is fatty liver. Ninety per cent of these patients have fatty infiltration of the liver preoperatively, but in almost half this may increase during the first year or two before regressing. During this period a few develop symptoms and signs of fatty liver (anorexia, nausea, and profound lethargy together with enlargement of the liver). Such patients need admission to hospital for parenteral nutrition and elemental diet. Failure to respond may necessitate reversal of the bypass, for this complication is the main cause of death. There is also a low incidence of cirrhosis.

The morbidity of small-bowel bypass has been stressed to emphasise that this procedure should not be considered lightly as the easy way out or as "the answer to the fatties' prayer." Equally, it must be recognised that most patients do extremely well, benefiting physically, psychiatrically, socially, and economically. The hazards mentioned may be reduced by better case selection, eliminating all patients with known heart disease, low intelligence, severe psychiatric disturbance, and alcoholism. But as the operation still remains to be evaluated in the long term it should be performed only on those who are in danger of succumbing to the complications of obesity.

Copies of diet sheets are available on request from Dr Bennett.

Index

Index

Index

Index

Index

Index

Index

Index

Index

Index

Index

Index